Essentials of Computed Tomography

Essentials of Computed Tomography

Dr. Roy George
MBBS, DNB RD, DMRD, MNAMS, MCCP
Consultant & Head, Deptt. of Imaging Sciences,
Century Hospital, Chengannur, Kerala - 689505
Presently Specialist in Radiology,
Hadi Hospital, Hawalli, Kuwait

CBS

CBS PUBLISHERS & DISTRIBUTORS
NEW DELHI • BANGALORE

ISBN : 81-239-1348-6

First Edition : 2006

Publishing Director : Vinod K. Jain

Published by :
Satish Kumar Jain for CBS Publishers & Distributors,
4596/1-A, 11 Darya Ganj, New Delhi - 110 002 (India)
E-mail: cbspubs@vsnl.com • Website: www.cbspd.com

Branch Office :
2975, 17th Cross, K.R. Road, Bansankari 2nd Stage, Bangalore-70
Fax : 080-26771680 • E-mail : cbsbng@vsnl.net

Printed at :
India Binding House, Noida (U.P.)

FOREWORD

Foreword

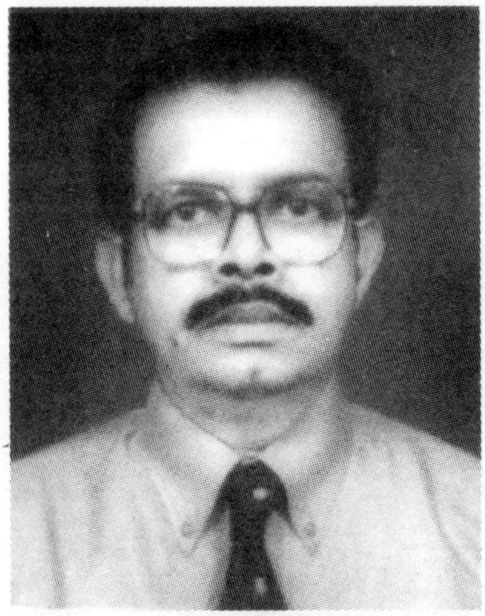

Dr. SUDHIR
MD, DMRD, FRCR
Professor and Head, Department of Radiodiagnosis,
Pushpagiri Medical College, Thiruvalla, Kerala

It is essential that those working in the discipline of medical imaging should at least be in the possesion of up-to-date basic knowledge. This requirement is met by this handbook **Essentials of Computed Tomography**. It provides a spectrum of knowledge as well.This book is intended to be brief and broad and thorough update of what every radiologist and technologist needs to know about CT imaging. I sincerely hope that this volume will be of help to students and radiologists and will be used extensively in all CT scan training centres. I congratulate Dr Roy on his maiden attempt.

PREFACE

Preface

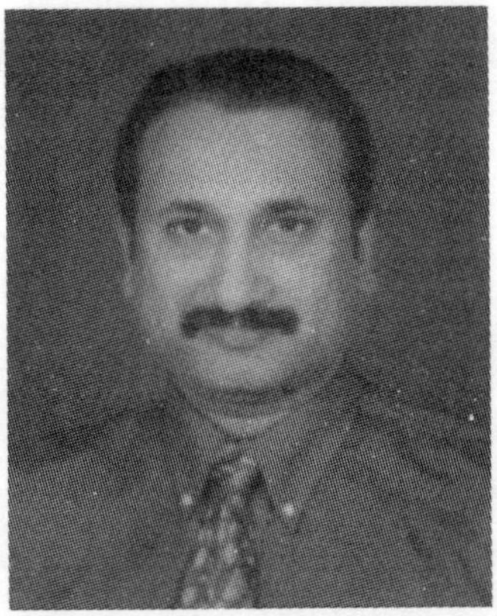

Computed tomography has been extensively used in clinical practice over the past many years. Even with the advent of magnetic resonance imaging into the fray, CT scans still remain the modality of choice for many diagnostic problems. Myriad technological developments were added on to enhance its utility as a composite and effective diagnostic tool. Several of these techniques e.g. spiral CT and multislice CT, even reversed the trend towards over-usage of MRI scans.

The day-to-day improvisation in the technological arena has challenged the radiologists and technologists inspiring them to cope up with the latest trends. To equip them to surpass this technological shock, imaging personnel need more comprehensive and clear understanding of the fundamental principles of CT imaging. The basic physical principles employed in the working of CT scans are the key areas of this book.

There are numerous conventional foreign-authored textbooks describing CT physics elaborately, but they find limited utility for our technologists because of the lack of brevity and unaffordable pricing. Most of the books available in India do not describe the evolution, generations, technological advancements, image manipulation and latest trends amply. This has stimulated me to get into a venture of bringing out a lucid handbook, that would be comprehensive.

The vast amount of literature has been painstakingly shrunken into a concise book without losing adequate information. I do hope that this book gives an overview of principles and clinical applications of computerized tomography that will surely aid the radiologists, students and staff radiographers. I have intentionally omitted many complicated formulae and calculations to keep up the brevity of the text.

I would like to extend my sincere thanks to Miss Razia Beevi, our technologist, who has taken lot of efforts in compiling the data and organizing the chapters. I appreciate Mr. Aji Pe my secretary for his sincere help in this venture. I would be glad if this book turns out to be a helpful guide for the postgraduates and technologists. Any constructive criticism or suggestions for improving the content are welcome.

Dr. ROY GEORGE

CONTENTS

Contents

CHAPTER

1 The History

The advent of X-rays in 1895 was an epoch-making achievement that ear-marked the progress in diagnostic and therapeutic radiology. X-rays are, by large, the most readily accessible, and commonly used imaging tool in the world. The limitation of plain radiographic techniques is the two-dimensional representation of a three-dimensional structure.

The word "tomography" can be traced back to early 1920s where investigators were developing techniques to image a specific section of the body. However, it was Grossman, who defined the technique and labeled it tomography in 1935. A conventional tomogram is an image of a section of the patient that is oriented parallel to the film. Watson in England (1937) developed another tomographic technique in which the sections were transverse sections (cross sections); and this technique was referred to as transverse axial tomography. These images, however, lacked adequate detail and clarity to be useful in diagnostic radiology, so the technique was not fully realized as a clinical tool.

"Computerized Tomography" overcomes these limitations by using a procedure known as image reconstruction from projections. Radiation passes through tissue in a specific way and is projected onto a detector that sends signals to a computer for processing. The computer produces clear, sharp images of the internal structure of the object. Hounsfield, in England, applied reconstruction techniques to produce the world's first clinically useful CT scanner for imaging the brain in 1967. He called the technique computerized transverse axial scanning (tomography) in 1973. Since then, a number of other terms have appeared in the literature. Terms such as computerized transverse axial tomography (CTAT), computer-assisted tomography (CAT), computerized transaxial transmission reconstructive tomography (CTTRT), and computerized tomography (CT) were not uncommon. The term "computed tomography" (CT) was established by the Radiological Society of North America through their major journal, "Radiology".

SCIENTISTS BEHIND CT

1. Godfrey Newbold Hounsfield

Godfrey Newbold Hounsfield was born in 1919 in England. He graduated in electrical and mechanical engineering in 1951 and joined at EMI (Electrical and Musical Industries). In 1967 he studied and concluded that by applying reconstruction techniques after X-ray beam were passed through an object from all directions and if measurements were made of all the X-ray transmissions it is possible to obtain information about internal structures. And further studies with Dr James Ambrose led to the invention of CT scanner. The first patient was scanned in 1972. He shared the Nobel Prize in medicine and physiology with Allan McLeod Cormack for their contributions in CT.

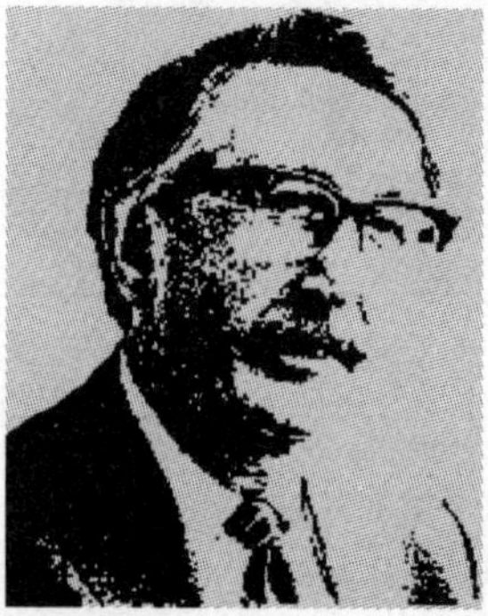

Fig. 1.1. Dr. Godfrey Hounsfield, inventor of CT.

2. Dr James Ambrose

A consultant radiologist at Atkinson-Morley's Hospital. He together with Hounsfield has done a lot of experiments on specimen of human brain. In 1971 the first clinical prototype CT brain scanner was installed in his hospital and clinical studies were conducted under his directions.

3. Allan McLeod Cormack

He was born in Johannesburg, South Africa in 1924. He studied nuclear physics at Cambridge University. Professor Cormack developed solutions to the mathematical problems involved in CT. He shared the Nobel Prize with Hounsfield for their contributions in CT.

THE MILESTONES

Year	Development	Inventor/Place
1895	X-ray was invented	William Conrad Roentgen
1935	Tomography	Grossman
1937	Transverse Axial Tomography	Watson
1967	Experiment towards CT	Godfrey Newbold Hounsfield.
1972	First patient was scanned by CT	In Atkinson-Morley's Hospital
1973	Paper on CT was published in BJR	Hounsfield

1972-74	First 3 generations of CT
1974	Fourth generation CT
1983-85	Fifth generation CT
1986	Osteo CT
1990	Spiral CT
1994	Sub-Second CT
1998	Multislice CT

CHAPTER 2

An Introduction to CT

INTRODUCTION

CT uses a computer to process information collected from the passage of X-ray beams through an area of anatomy. The images created are cross sectional. To help the beginner to visualize CT, the loaf of bread analogy is useful. If the patient's body is imagined to be a loaf of bread, the crust of the bread is analogous to the skin of the patient's body, and the white portion of bread relates to the patient's internal organs. Each CT slice represents a specific plane in the patient's body. The thickness of the plane is referred to as its Z-axis. The Z-axis determines the thickness of the slices. The data that forms the CT slice are further sectioned in two elements: X indicates Width, and Y indicates Height.

Each one of these two-dimensional squares is a pixel (picture element) on the CT monitor. The CT image is a composite of pixels for each slice. If the X-axis is taken into account, the result is a cube, rather than a square. This cube is referred to as a voxel. A matrix is a grid formed from the rows and columns of pixels. Although some scanners have a matrix size of 1024, the most common matrix size is 512. This size translates to 512 rows of pixels down and 512 columns of pixels across. The total number of pixels present in a

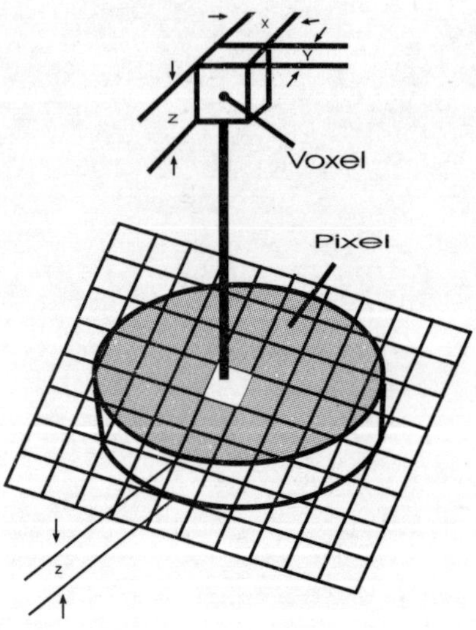

Fig. 2.1. Graphic representaion of pixel and voxel.

matrix is the product of the number of rows and number of columns, in this case 512 × 512. Each pixel contains information that the computer obtains from scanning.

The formation of CT images by a CT scanner involves a three-step process which involves :

1. Data acquisition
2. Data processing
3. Image display, manipulation, recording and storage.

I. DATA ACQUISITION

The term "data acquisition" refers to the systematic collection of x-ray transmission measurements from the patient to produce the CT image. Once x-rays have passed through the patient, they fall on to special detectors that measure the transmission values (attenuation values). There are two methods of data acquisition

1. Slice-by-slice data acquisition
2. Volume data acquisition.

In conventional slice-by-slice data acquisition, data are collected using a number of different beam geometries to scan the patient. Essentially, the x-ray tube rotates around the patient and collects data from the first slice. The tube comes to a stop and the patient is moved into position so that the next slice can be scanned. This process continues until all slices have been scanned, one slice at a time. In volume data acquisition, a special beam geometry referred to as spiral or helical geometry is used to scan a volume of tissue rather than one slice at a time. In spiral CT, the x-ray tube rotates around the patient and traces a spiral (helical) path to scan an entire volume of tissue during a single breath hold. During scanning, the x-ray tube and detectors rotate around the patient to collect views. From a number of different locations, the detectors measure the radiation transmitted through the patient from all these different locations. As a result, relative transmission values or penetration measurements can be calculated:

$$\text{Relative transmission} = \log \frac{\text{Intensity of x-rays at the source } (I_0)}{\text{Intensity of x-rays at the detector } (I)}$$

The relative transmission values are sent to the computer and stored as raw data.

II. DATA PROCESSING

Data processing essentially constitutes the mathematical principles involved in CT. The computer uses special mathematical techniques to reconstruct the CT image in a finite number of steps called reconstruction algorithms.

Transmission values collected as a result of scanning the patient are stored as raw data in the computer. In CT, data processing is a three-step process. First the raw data undergoes some form of preprocessing in which corrections are made and some reformatting of the data takes place. This is necessary to facilitate the next step in data processing, image reconstruction. The scan data, which represent penetration measurements, are converted into a digital image characterized by numbers called CT numbers. These numbers are related to the linear attenuation coefficients. Conversion of the transmission measurements into a CT image is accomplished by mathematical procedures referred to as reconstruction techniques or reconstruction algorithms. Several reconstruction techniques have been developed; these include simple back-projection, iterative methods, and analytic methods.

III. IMAGE MANIPULATION, DISPLAY, RECORDING AND STORAGE

Once the computer has performed the image reconstruction process, the constructed image can be displayed and recorded for subsequent viewing, as well as stored for re-analysis at some later time.

Image manipulation

In image manipulation, images can be modified to make them more useful to the observer. For example, transverse images can be reformatted into coronal, sagittal, and paraxial sections. In addition, images can also be subjected to other image processing operations, such as image smoothing, edge enhancement, gray scale manipulation, and three-dimensional processing etc.

Image display

Once the CT image has been reconstructed by the computer it exists in digital form. This must be converted to a form that is not only suitable for viewing but also meaningful to the observer. In CT, the digital reconstructed image is converted into a gray scale image for interpretation by the radiologist. The gray scale image is displayed on a cathode ray tube (CRT), or television monitor, which is an essential component of the control or viewing console.

Image recording

Images are usually recorded on x-ray film. Such recording is accomplished by multiformat video cameras, but laser cameras have been developed and are now very common. Dry laser cameras are slowly getting introduced into the field.

Image storage

Image storage refers to storage of the reconstructed digital images. The digital image is held in a disk memory for short-term storage. They also can be stored on magnetic tapes and magnetic disks. More recently, optical storage technology has added a new dimension to the storage of information from CT scanners.

IV. SEQUENCE OF EVENTS

The sequence of events can be summarized as follows:

The x-ray tube rotates around the patient, who is positioned in the gantry aperture for the CT examination. This is the first step in the data acquisition process, which is characterized by the beam geometry and method of scanning, and that involves passing x-rays through the patient. The x-ray beam is highly collimated by pre-patient collimators. As the radiation passes through the patient, it is attenuated. The detectors measure the transmitted photons.

The transmitted beam and the reference beam are both converted into electrical current signals that undergo amplification by special circuits. This is followed by logarithmic amplification, in which the relative transmission readings are changed into attenuation and thickness data. Before the data are sent to the computer, they must be converted into digital form. The digital data undergo some form of preprocessing which includes corrections and reformatting. The preprocessed data are referred to as reformatted raw data. Additional data corrections are performed on the data using computer software.

Convolution is performed on the data after various corrections by the array of processors. A special algorithm is then used to reconstruct an image of the internal anatomic structures being examined. This is the back-projection reconstruction algorithm. The reconstructed image can then be displayed, it can be recorded on film using a laser camera, or it can be stored on magnetic or optical tape and/or disks. The image processor allows for various image-processing operations to be performed on the displayed image.

CHAPTER 3 Data Acquisition in CT

I. INTRODUCTION

Data acquisition in CT refers to the method by which the patient is scanned, and obtains enough data for image reconstruction. Scanning is defined by the beam geometry, which not only characterizes the particular CT system, but also plays a central role in spatial resolution and artifact production. The term "beam geometry" refers to the geometric properties of the x-ray beam (e.g., size and shape) from the x-ray tube to the detectors. It encompasses collimation and, more importantly, the systematic motion of the beam as it scans the patient to acquire x-ray transmission data.

2. BASIC STEPS

The basic steps of data acquisition can be described as follows. The x-ray tube and detector are in perfect alignment. The tube and detector move around the patient to collect a large number of transmission measurements during each scan. As the beam leaves the tube, a special filter shapes it. The beam is then collimated to pass through only the slice of interest. The beam is attenuated by the patient and the detector then measures the transmitted photons. The detector converts the x-ray photons into an electrical signal (analog data). These signals are then converted by the detector electronics, the analog-to-digital converter (ADC), into digital data. The digital data are sent to the computer for image reconstruction.

3. DATA ACQUISITION GEOMETRIES

There are three primary types of acquisition geometries. These have been described as parallel beam geometry, fan beam geometry, and CT scanning in spiral geometry. As a result, a simple categorization of CT equipment has evolved based on the scanning geometry, scanning motion, and the number of detectors.

4. FIRST-GENERATION SCANNERS : PARALLEL BEAM GEOMETRY (TRANSLATE-ROTATE)

First-generation scanner, is based on the parallel beam geometry and the translate-rotate scanning motion. A single, highly collimated x-ray beam and one or two detectors first translate across the patient and collect transmission readings. After one translation, the tube and detector rotate by 1^0 and translate once again, collecting readings from a different direction. This is done for 180^0 around the patient. Scan times were very long in this model. Parallel beam geometry was first used by Hounsfield in his original experiments in CT. The first EMI brain scanner, as well as earlier scanners (built by other manufacturers), were based on this concept. This design is no longer in use. First-generation CT scanners took at least 3-5 minutes to produce a complete scan of the patient, a major limitation that placed a restriction on patient throughput.

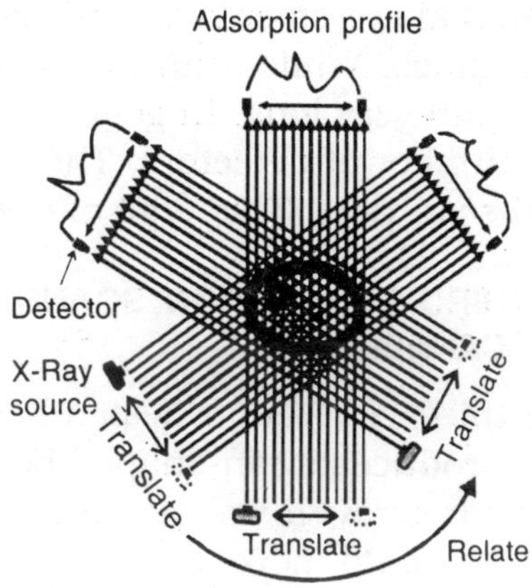

Fig 3.1. 1st Generation CT

5. SECOND-GENERATION SCANNER : FAN BEAM GEOMETRY: (TRANSLATE-ROTATE)

The second-generation design is one in which the x-ray beam also passed linearly across the patient before rotating. However, a fan-shaped x-ray beam was used, rather than the thin beam used with first generation designs. Only part of the field of view could be covered with this fan beam. These were also based on the translate-rotate principle of first-generation machines, with a few fundamentally different features. Two of these include a linear detector array coupled to the x-ray tube and multiple pencil beams, with each individual beam falling on one detector. The result of this is a beam geometry that describes a small fan, in which the apex of the fan originates at the x-ray tube. This is the fan beam geometry. An important characteristic of fan beam geometry is that the rays constituting the fan are now divergent instead of

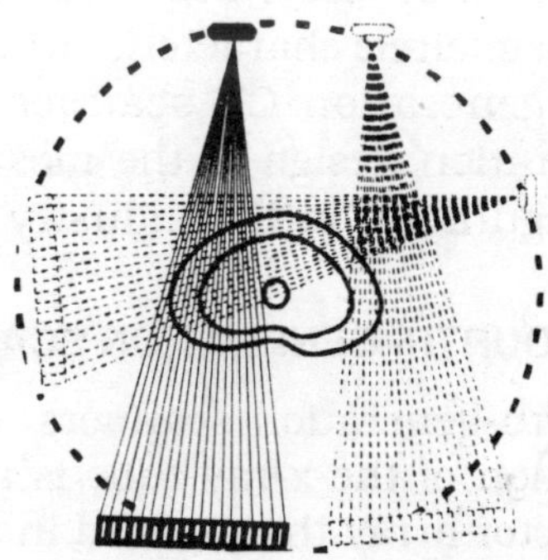

Fig. 3.2. 2nd Generation CT Scanner.

parallel. This results in a significant change in the image reconstruction algorithm, which must be capable of handling projection data from the fan beam geometry. The fan beam translates across the patient to collect a set of transmission readings. After one translation, the tube and detector array rotate by larger increments and translate once again. This process is repeated for 180° and is referred to as rectilinear multiple pencil beam scanning. The larger rotational increments and the increased number of detectors result in shorter scan times. While scan times were shorter than in the original design, they were still very long. In general, the time decrease is inversely proportional to the number of detectors. The more the number of detectors, the shorter the total scan time. This type of design is also no longer in use.

6. THIRD-GENERATION SCANNERS FAN BEAM GEOMETRY (ROTATE-ROTATE SCANNERS)

The third generation design consists of a detector array and an x-ray tube that produces a fan-shaped beam that covered the entire field of view and a detector array. It was no longer necessary to translate the beam and detector as both could move in a circle within the gantry. The rotating detector design allows all of the readings that make up a view to be recorded instantaneously and simultaneously. This greatly reduced scan times. These are sometimes referred to as rotate-rotate scanners. Third-generation CT scanners are based on the use of fan beam geometry, which rotates continuously around the patient for 360°. The x-ray tube is coupled to a curved detector array that subtends an arc of about 30° to 40° from the apex of the fan located at the x-ray tube. As the x-ray tube and detectors rotate, projection profiles are collected and, for every fixed point of the tube and detector, a view is obtained. This motion is referred to as continuously rotating fan beam scanning. The path traced by the tube describes a circle rather than the semicircle characteristic of first and second-generation CT scanners. The third-generation design is the most widely used configuration in the industry today.

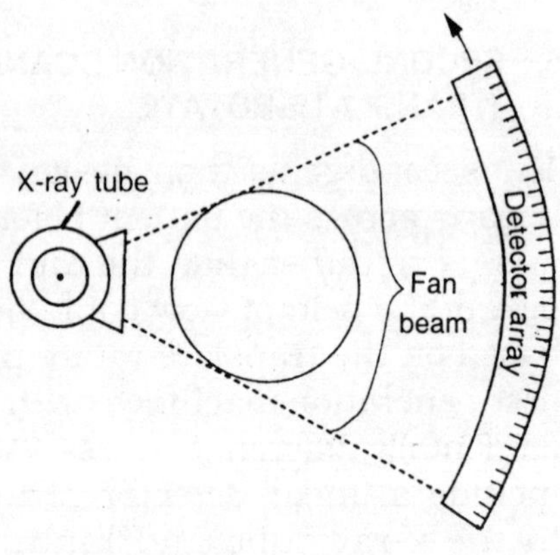

Fig. 3.3. Third Generation Scanner.

7. FOURTH–GENERATION SCANNERS : FAN BEAM GEOMETRY (ROTATE-NONE)

Fourth-generation scanners are based on fan beam geometry and complete rotation of the x-ray tube is around a stationary ring of detectors. It uses a detector array that is fixed in a 360° circle within the gantry. The tube rotates within the fixed detector array and produces a fan-shaped beam. However, the number of detectors in use at any one time is controlled by the width of the beam. In the stationary detector design, the readings that make up a view are recorded consecutively over approximately one-fifth of the scan time. Fourth generation scanners are also called rotate-none systems. The x-ray tube is positioned within a stationary, circular detector array. The beam geometry describes a wide fan. The apex of the fan now originates at each of the detectors – that is, each detector position gives rise to a fan. As the tube moves from point to point within the circle, single rays strike a detector from point to point. In this way, view is obtained. Scan times are very short and vary from scanner to scanner, depending on the manufacturer. The path traced by the x-ray tube is circular. The image reconstruction algorithm is for a fan beam geometry, in which the apex of the fan is now at the detector, as opposed to the x-ray tube in the third-generation systems.

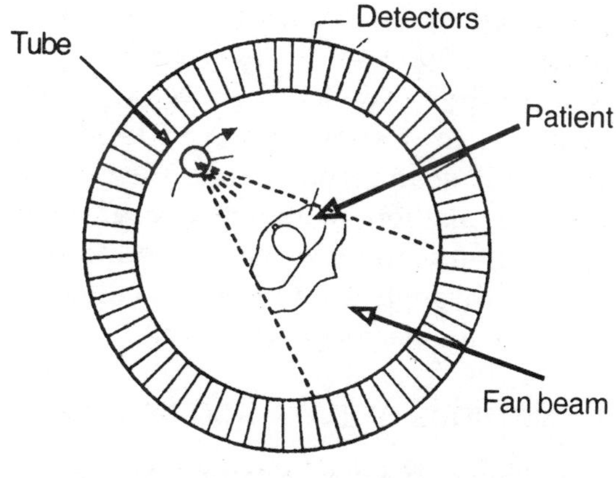

Fig. 3.4. 4th Generation CT Scanner

8. FIFTH GENERATION SCANNERS : ELECTRON BEAM GEOMETRY

Fifth-generation scanners developed primarily for what has come to be known as high-speed CT scanning. These scanners are based on special configurations intended to facilitate very fast scanning. This system that was originally

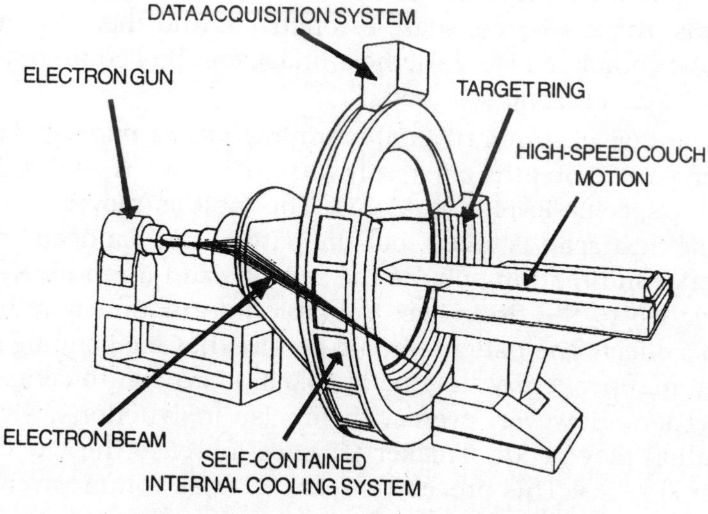

Fig. 3.5. 5th Generation CT Scanner

produced by Imatron, uses a large electron gun as its x-ray beam source. A massive anode target is placed in a semicircular ring around the patient. Neither the x-ray beam source nor the detectors move, and the scans can be acquired in a short time. Fifth-generation scanners are classified as high-speed CT scanners because they can acquire scan data in milliseconds. The data acquisition geometry is a fan beam. X-rays produced by a beam of electrons that scans over several stationary tungsten target rings. The fan beam passes through the patient to collect the x-ray transmission readings necessary for image reconstruction.

9. METHODS OF DATA ACQUISITION

A. STANDARD AXIAL AQUISITION

This method is the oldest and most widely used means of collecting data. It consists of (1) having the patient in suspended respiration (for body scans), (2) acquiring data for a single slice, (3) allowing the patient to resume normal breathing, (4) moving the table to the next slice location, and (5) repeating the procedure until the desired area is covered. Historically, all scanners were designed to function this way. New scanners still can function in a standard axial mode if desired. Scanners that function exclusively in this manner do so for a number of reasons. First, time is required for an x-ray tube to rotate in one direction, stop, and then rotate in the opposite direction. Generally, a patient can only hold his breath for one rotation of the x-ray tube. Second, a system may require the tube to cool before another scan can be obtained. This tube cooling takes 3 to 30 seconds. The patient must be allowed to breath while the tube cools. Third, some scanner systems do not permit sequential scans to be obtained while the computer reconstructs images and displays them. That is, these systems scan, reconstruct, and then display. The entire cycle must be complete before the next image can be acquired. Such systems are referred to as pipeline scanners.

A disadvantage of standard axial scanning is **slice misregistration,** which occurs when patient breaths differently with each scan. A shallow breath places the slice at a specific level of anatomy. The table is moved to the next scan position. The next scan is taken, but the patient takes a deep breath instead. This difference in breathing places the second scan in an incorrect anatomic position relative to the first slice. Valuable information may be missed because of this effect. The patient should be told that suspending respiration in an identical manner, every time he is asked, is crucial to completing a quality examination. However, even with precise instructions, significant slice misregistration may occur. Thicker CT slice increase the likelihood of missing very small areas. This process is referred to as volume averaging, or **Partial volume effect**. Volume average occurs when different tissues are averaged together. This phenomenon results in missing and misinterpretation of lesions.

B. NON-INCREMENTAL CT (Single location sequential studies)

The term **Dynamic scanning** is confusing and this term is rapidly becoming obsolete. It has different meanings to different people. Early scanners often had interscan delay time of 30 seconds or more. Often, scanning within peak contrast enhancement was impossible because of these delays. Because of this disadvantage, dynamic scanning was born. In the truest sense of the word, dynamic scan refers to slices that are performed at a speed faster than the system's usual mode. This procedure is often accomplished by lowering the milliampere-second (mAs) level to reduce tube cooling time. On some scanners, it is possible to suspend image reconstructions and therefore speed up scan acquisition. The liver is the most common organ selected for dynamic scanning. In this way, the liver can be scanned at peak contrast enhancement. Dynamic scanning is often used in the diagnosis of liver hemangiomas. For these applications, it is necessary to scan repeatedly at the same table position. This type of scanning is done to evaluate the enhancement of the suspected hemangioma. Because of its common use in this manner, many practitioners incorrectly define dynamic scanning as rapid scanning done at the same level of anatomy. Because new scanners are much faster, often performing routine scans faster than those once called dynamic, the term is becoming obsolete. In its place are the terms rapid acquisition scanning and rapid scan. If the scanning is done at the same level of anatomy, the descriptive term is nonincremental scanning.

TYPES OF NON-INCREMENTAL SCANNING

1. Continuous data acquisition
2. Intermittent data acquisition

1. Continuous data acquisition

Continuous non-incremental acquisition of data from a single location opens considerable avenues for physiological and pathophysiological studies. It also allows transit of contrast evaluation in structures with rapid flow. Although such physiological studies are better performed with an ultrafast electron gun CT, it can be evaluated by spiral CT machines.

2. Intermittent data acquisition

This may be used for slower events. It reduces the radiation dose to the site also. Respiratory misregistration is a problem. This approach may be inappropriate when evaluating a small lesion.

A. **Morphologic information** : Example: Hepatic hemangioma

Scan timing can be 20 sec, 30 sec, 50 sec, 60 sec, 100 sec, 120 sec, etc. An optional evaluation would be short initial continuous data acquisition and a subsequent series of intermittent exposure.

B. **Functional information :** The way in which tissues take up contrast media at CT can be used to assess function (Perfusion). Series of exposures at certain interval after a bolus injection and by means of software which allows pixel by pixel calculation, colour maps of perfusion can be generated and in some instances these can make lesion more obvious.

C. CLUSTER SCANNING

Cluster scanning is the practice of grouping more than one scan in a single breath hold. Grouping scans in this way is possible because newer scanners are much faster than their predecessors. The number of scans is dependent on how long the patient can hold his/her breath. The primary advantage of this method of scanning is the reduction in slice misregistration. Another benefit is decreased examination time. A disadvantage of scanning at increased speed is that image reconstruction cannot keep up with data acquisition. Therefore, the image displayed on the monitor can lag significantly behind the slice that is being taken. The routine of watching images as they appear and making adjustments accordingly is not practical when scanning at this increased rate.

D. CONTINUOUS ACQUISITION SCANNING (SPIRAL/HELICAL)

Scanners that offer the option of spiral scanning are also capable of producing scans with the traditional axial method. The spiral method uses a continually rotating x-ray gantry with constant x-ray output and uninterrupted table movement. Because the data are acquired continually as opposed to the start-and-stop method used in conventional axial scanning; the result is a volume, or block, of data. Acquiring a volume of information allows images to be manipulated in ways not available with conventional acquisition method. Although the result is a block of data, it is important to remember that this information is acquired in thin ribbons, not one block at a time. Numerous advancements make this technology possible. Although virtually indistinguishable in appearance, the images produced by this method are not precisely axial. An axial image is taken so that each slice is parallel to every other slice, like bangles on a wrist. With a spiral technique, the images are similar to a spring, with each slice at a slight angle. In general, to offer a higher range of milliampere settings, it is necessary to increase both the size of the generator and the tube cooling capabilities of the system. These modifications significantly increase the cost of the CT system. Slowing the tube rotation from 1 to 2 seconds doubles the milliampere-second level. Obviously, examination time will also be increased.

CHAPTER 4

Digital Image Processing

1. ANALOG VERSUS DIGITAL IMAGE

Analog images are continuous images, for example, a chest x-ray. Digital images, on the other hand, are numerical representations of objects or images of objects. The formation of digital images requires a digital computer. Any information that goes to the computer for processing must first be converted into digital form (numbers). An important component is the analog-to-digital converter (ADC), which changes continuous signals into discrete signals (digital data). In processing an image, it is necessary to convert an input image into an output image. If the input image is analog in nature and the output image is also analog, this is referred to as analog processing. On the other hand, if the input image is discrete and the output image is also discrete, this is referred to as digital processing. In cases in which the analog image must be converted into digital data for input to the computer, a digitization system is required. Digital image processing can be defined as "subjecting numerical representations of objects to a series of operations in order to obtain a desired result".

2. DIGITIZING AN IMAGE

The primary objective when digitizing an image is to convert an analog image into numerical data for processing by the computer, a conversion process known as digitization. The process of digitization consists of three distinct steps :

1. Scanning
2. Sampling
3. Quantization

Scanning : The first step in digitization is division of the picture into small regions, a process known as scanning. Each small region of the picture is called a picture element, or pixel. The result of scanning is a grid characterized by rows and columns. The size of the grid usually depends on the number of pixels on each side of grid. The rows and columns play a role in identifying a particular pixel by providing an "address" for that pixel. The rows and columns make up what has been referred to as a matrix.

Sampling : The second step in digitizing an image is sampling, a procedure done on the entire image in which the brightness of each pixel is measured. A small spot of light is projected onto the transparency and a photomultiplier tube positioned behind the picture detects the transmitted light. The output of the photomultiplier tube is an electrical signal (analog signal).

Quantization : Quantization is the final step in digitizing a picture. In quantization, the brightness value of each pixel sampled is assigned an integer (0, or a positive or negative number) called a gray level. This is done for all the pixels that make up the picture and the result is a range of numbers or gray levels, each of which has a precise location on the rectangular grid of pixels. The total number of gray levels is called the gray scale. In quantization, the electrical signal is assigned an integer based on the strength of the signal. In general, the value of the integer is proportional to the signal strength. At the end of the quantization process we have a digital image, an array of numbers representing the analog image that we scanned, sampled, and quantized. This array of numbers is sent to the computer for further processing.

3. ADVANTAGES OF DIGITIZATION

The major goal of digitization is that a computer can process digital images.

Some of the major advantages of digitalisation are mentioned below :

1. **Image Enhancement:** The image can be made to look more pleasing to the observer. Certain characteristics of the image, such as contours and shapes, can be enhanced to improve the overall quality of the image.
2. **Image Restoration:** Poor images can be filtered to remove unwanted "noise", a technique referred to as filtering. Filtering can also help to remove unnecessary fine detail in the image, a technique known as smoothing.
3. **Image Analysis:** This is also referred to as scene analysis, which "seeks to extract the information contained in the various objects in a scene without placing any interpretation on them".
4. **Image Detection**: The advantage of detection is to allow the observer to look for specific shapes, contours, or textures while disregarding the other features in the image.
5. **Pattern Recognition:** In digital image processing, the computer can "see" structures and identify patterns.

6. **Geometric Transformation:** In this process, images can be rotated or scaled by changing the position of the pixels.
7. **Data Compression:** The compression of digital images reduces the amount of data that make up the image. This is important when the data has to be stored or transmitted.

4. CT AS A DIGITAL IMAGE PROCESSING SYSTEM

As a digital image processing system, CT fits into this scheme. Similar steps in digitizing an image can be applied to the CT process. In digitizing an image, the first step is to divide up the picture into small regions, called pixels. In CT, the slice of the patient to be examined is essentially divided into small regions called voxels because the dimension of depth (slice thickness) is added to the pixel. In CT, this is done by scanning the patient with the x-ray tube moving around the patient. The second step in digitizing a picture is to sample the pixels. In CT, the voxels are sampled when x-rays pass through them. Detectors do this measurement. At this point, it is also important to realize that the signal coming from the detector is an analog signal, which must be converted into digital form before it can be sent to the computer for processing. This means that the analog signal has to be sampled by the ADC. The final step in digitizing a picture is quantization. In CT, the analog signal is also quantized and changed into a digital array for input into the computer. In digitizing an image, the digital data are processed by the computer using a series of image processing operations or techniques to modify the input image. In CT, the digital data are also subject to several processing algorithms, so that the output image can be displayed in a form suitable for viewing by a human observer.

CHAPTER 5

Data Processing (Image Reconstruction)

I. INTRODUCTION TO BASIC PRINCIPLES AND TERMINOLOGY

Image reconstruction from projections is "the process of producing an image of a two-dimensional distribution from estimates of its line integrals along with a finite number of lines of known locations. In describing the mathematics of CT, it is important to understand the basic principles related to the image reconstruction process. These include algorithms, Fourier transformation, convolution and interpolation.

Ray sum and view

The path that the x-ray beam takes from the tube to the detector is referred to as a ray. The detector reads each arriving ray and measures how much of the beam is attenuated. This measurement is called a ray sum. A complete set of ray sums is known as a view. A view is similar to a person looking at an object. From only one angle, it is difficult to obtain a true understanding of the shape of the object. To obtain the most realistic picture of the object, it would be best to walk around and observe it from many angles. The observer's final evaluation of the object would involve all of his observations. The CT image is created in much the same way. Multiple views are needed to create an image.

Attenuation profile

The system accounts for the attenuation properties of each ray sum and correlates them with the position of the ray. The result of this type of correlation is called an attenuation profile.

Back projection

An attenuation profile is created for each view in the scan. The information from all of the profiles is projected onto a matrix. This process of converting the data from the attenuation profile to a matrix is known as back projection.

Convolution

There is a significant drawback in projecting data onto a matrix; it produces streaks, or artifacts, on the image. To minimize the artifacts caused by back projection a process called **filtering** is applied to the scanned data before back projection occurs. The process of applying a filter function to an attenuation profile is called **convolution**. Convolution is a digital image processing technique. It is intended to modify images through the use of a filter function. "The process involves multiplication of overlapping portions of the filter function and the detector response curve selectively to produce a third function which is used for image reconstruction."

Hard disk and storage

Each time the x-ray is activated, information is gathered and fed into the system computer. The computer processes thousands of bits of data from each scan acquired and saved on a computer file so that the information will be available for use in the formation of an image. These stored data can later be retrieved and manipulated. The hard disk is the device within the computer that saves this information. The hard disk is an essential component of all CT systems. The number of images that the hard disk can store varies according to the make and model of the scanner. It is important to remember that an enormous amount of information is collected for each image. For example, a single image in a 512 matrix system consists of 262,144 pixels (512 × 512). The digitization requires 10 to 12 bits; an 8-bit byte is standard. Therefore, it takes 2 bytes to cover each pixel in the dynamic range. This requirement translates to 2 × 262,144 = 524,288 bytes, or 0.52 megabytes (MB). When a 1024 matrix system is used, each image requires approximately 2 MB.

Raw data

All of the thousands of bits of data acquired by the system with each scan are called raw data. The terms scan data and raw data are used interchangeably to refer to the data sitting in the computer and waiting to be made into an image.

Image data

To form an image, the computer assigns one value (HU) to each pixel. This value, or density number, is the average of all measurements for that pixel. The two-dimensional pixel represents a three-dimensional portion of patient tissue. The pixel value represents the proportional amount of x-ray energy that passes through anatomy and strikes the detector. Once the data are averaged so that each pixel has one associated number, an image can be formed. The data included in this image are appropriately called image data. Image data require approximately one-fifth of the computer space needed for raw data. For this reason, CT systems may allow space for 3000 image data files, but only 350 raw data files. If only the image data are available, data manipulation is limited. Image data allow measurements such as Hounsfield units, standard deviation and distance, but anything not seen on the image is unavailable for analysis.

Image reconstruction

The process of using raw data to create an image is called image reconstruction. The reconstruction that is automatically produced during scanning is often called prospective reconstruction. The same raw data may be used later to generate a new image. This process is referred to as retrospective reconstruction.

Scan field of view

Scan field of view is also called calibration field of view. Selecting the scan field of view determines the area, within the gantry, from which the raw data are acquired. Because scan data are always acquired around the isocenter, the patient must be positioned in the center of the gantry. Scan field of view selection determines the number of detector cells collecting data. The choices of scan field of view vary among scanners. Typical choices are small (25 cm), which is used for the head; medium (35 cm), which is often used for the chest; and large (40–50 cm), which is used for the abdomen. Anything outside the scan field of view circle is not imaged because no data are collected beyond this circle. To produce the highest quality image, the operator should select the scan field of view that comes closer to just encompassing the patient. It is important that no part of the patient lies outside the scan field. Part of the patient located outside the scan field may cause inaccuracies in the image, called **out-of-field artifacts.** These artifacts cause streaking, shading and incorrect Hounsfield numbers. Selecting the correct scan field of view is important to reduce out-of-field artifacts. Selecting too large a display field makes the image appear unnecessarily small.

Display field of view

Selecting the display field of view determines how much of the raw data are used to create an image. For example, if a lumbar spine is correctly scanned with a large scan field of view to include the entire body, but the operator chooses to target the image so that the vertebrae occupy most of the screen, the rest of the patient's abdomen is not visualized on the image. The section that is visualized is the display field of view. Increasing the display field of view increases the size of each pixel within the image. Because more information is packed into each pixel, a loss of resolution can result. The display field of view and the matrix determine the pixel size. The size of the pixel can be determined by dividing the field of view by the matrix size.

$$\text{Pixel size} = \frac{\text{Field of view}}{\text{Matrix size}}$$

$$\text{Field of view} = \text{Pixel size} \times \text{Matrix size.}$$

It is important to understand that changing the display field of view does not distort the resulting image. To summarize, targeted reconstruction (i.e. adjusting the field of view size) allows the operator to match the scanner resolution to pixel size. Magnification will only make the image larger.

Kilovolt-peak setting

Increasing the kilovolt peak setting increases the intensity of the x-ray beam and the beam's ability to penetrate a thick, dense anatomic part. It may also decrease beam-hardening artifacts because of the increase in the average photon energy. If higher kilovolt-peak settings are available, they are typically recommended for use in the posterior fossa and lumbar spine.

Slice thickness

In general, thinner slices produce sharper images. The greater the slice thickness, the more pronounced the inaccuracies, particularly in tissue that is heterogeneous. This effect is called volume averaging or partial volume effect. Although the benefits of using thin slices in reducing volume averaging are considerable, there are significant drawbacks as well. Longer examination time, greater tube wear, use of more film and higher associated costs. Thin slices are used when the part being examined is small. A narrower beam produces a smaller number of detected photons. Therefore, the milliampere-second level must increase as slice thickness decreases. If the milliampere-second level is not adjusted to compensate for the thinner slice, resulting images will have a grainy, or noisy, appearance.

II. ALGORITHMS

An algorithm is "a set of rules or directions for getting a specific output from a specific input. The distinguishing feature of an algorithm is that all vagueness must be eliminated; the rules must describe operations that are so simple and well defined that they can be executed by a machine. Furthermore, an algorithm must always terminate after a finite number of steps". The solutions to mathematical problems in CT require that computer programs be used to reconstruct the image. These programs are referred to as **reconstruction algorithms**. The process of filtering data is often called convolution. Each algorithm uses a different mathematical formula for processing data. This formula enhances certain features of the CT image. In general, high contrast (also called bone, edge, detail, or sharp) algorithms are used to visualize structures with intrinsically high subject contrast, such as temporal bone or lung tissue. "Soft" algorithms are usually preferable for examining low contrast areas, such as the brain and abdomen. By using saved raw data, the same data can be retrospectively reconstructed into many images, each with a different algorithm. In a side-by-side comparison, it is much easier to determine which algorithm is best for a given application.

III. INTERPOLATION

Interpolation has been applied to the image reconstruction process, and to the determination of slices in spiral CT imaging. Interpolation is a mathematical technique used to estimate the value of a function from known values on either side of it. If known values of one variable, Y, are plotted against the other variable X, an estimate of an unknown value of Y can be made by drawing a straight line between the two nearest known values. Since the slice beginning does not match the slice end, each rotation is at a slight angle in spiral CT. Computer software adjusts for the slight angle by averaging the data and creating an image that is not slanted. Interpolation is the software technique applied here. The interpolation techniques improve longitudinal resolution. 180° interpolation result in increased longitudinal resolution as compared with 360° interpolation although at the expense of increased noise The three important advantages of 180° interpolation over 360° interpolation are that higher pitch can be used, reduced effective slice thickness and better longitudinal resolution.

IV. RECONSTRUCTION ALGORITHMS

1. Back projection

Back-projection also referred to as the summation method or linear superposition method. Consider four beams of x-rays passing through an unknown object to produce four projections, P_1, P_2, P_3, and P_4. The problem involves using these profiles to reconstruct an image of the unknown object. The projected data sets are back-projected to form the corresponding images BP_1; BP_2, BP_3 and BP_4. The reconstruction involves summing all these back-projected images to form an image of the object. The problem with the back-projection technique is that it does not produce a sharp image of the object and therefore is not used in clinical CT. The most striking artifact of back-projection is that of the typical "star" pattern, which occurs because points outside a high-density object receive some of the back-projected intensity of that object.

2. Iterative algorithms

An iterative reconstruction starts with an assumption and compares this assumption with measured values, makes corrections to bring the two into agreement, and then repeats this process over and over until the assumed and measured values are the same or within acceptable limits." These include the Simultaneous Iterative Reconstruction Technique (SIRT), Iterative Least-Squares Technique (ILST) and Algebraic Reconstruction Technique (ART). These techniques differ in the way in which corrections are applied to subsequent iterations. Hounsfield used the ART in the first EMI brain scanner.

3. Analytic reconstruction algorithms

Analytic reconstruction algorithms have been developed to overcome the limitations of the back-projection and iterative algorithms. They are used in modern CT scanners and have sound mathematical bases. The two analytic reconstruction algorithms are the Fourier reconstruction algorithm and filtered back-projection.

A. Filtered back-projection

Filtered back-projection is also referred to as the **convolution method.** It is similar to back-projection. The striking difference between the two is that the projection profile (data) is filtered or convoluted to remove the typical "star-like" blurring characteristic of the simple back-projection technique. Filtering is accomplished by convolution, which removes the blurring arising from back-projection with convolution.

B. Fourier transformation (FT)

In radiology the FT is used to reconstruct images of a patient's anatomy in CT. The FT is a mathematical function that converts a signal in the spatial domain to a signal in the frequency domain. The FT is a mathematical procedure for breaking down a waveform into a series of sine and cosine functions of different frequencies and amplitudes. By using Fourier coefficients it is possible to reconstruct an image in CT. A radiograph can be considered as an image in the spatial domain, that is, shades of gray represent various parts of the anatomy in space. By using the Fourier transformation this spatial domain image, the radiograph represented by the function f(x, y), can be transformed into the frequency domain to form a frequency domain image represented by the function F(u, v). This frequency domain image consists of frequencies ranging from high to low. In addition, this image can be transformed back into a spatial domain image by using the inverse Fourier transformation; there are several advantages to transforming a spatial domain image into a frequency domain image.

1. First, the image in the frequency domain can be manipulated by changing the amplitudes of the frequency components.
2. Second, a computer can be used to perform those manipulations. This leads to digital image processing.

3. The third advantage is that frequency information can be used to measure image quality through the use of the point spread function, line spread function, and modulation transfer function.

3D algorithms

Three-dimensional imaging uses 3D surface and volumetric reconstruction. The algorithms for 3D imaging are based on those used in such fields as computer graphics and visual perceptions science. An algorithm for surface display is based on at least two processes, preprocessing and display, and consists of the following four operations: interpolation, segmentation, surface formation, and projection.

Comparison of reconstruction algorithms

Essentially, analytic methods, filtered back-projection and the Fourier reconstruction, are faster and generate more accurate images than those obtained using iterative algorithms.

CHAPTER 6

Image Manipulation and Storage

I. DEFINITION

Those techniques (operations) or process which modify an image or group of images to enhance the visibility of useful information while suppressing 'noise' or non-useful information is called as image manipulation. An important point to note about image manipulation is that the operations do not produce any additional information. As a result "the information content in the processed image is always less than or equal to that in the original image".

II. TECHNIQUES

Image manipulation techniques fall into two major categories; linear and nonlinear techniques. Whereas linear techniques include such processes as image smoothing and enhancement, nonlinear techniques deal with gray scale manipulation, in which the gray scale of the image can be modified using different algorithms.

III. WINDOWING IN CT

Windowing refers to a method by which the CT image gray scale can be manipulated using the CT numbers that make up the image. The operator, to provide an optimum demonstration of the different structures seen on an image, can alter these numbers. There are more than 4000 different Hounsfield values; the monitor can display only 256 shades of gray. The human eye can differentiate only approximately 20 shades of gray.

Window width (WW) and Window level (WL)

The absorption measurement range in CT (expressed in Hounsfield units, or HU) is referred to as the **window width** (WW). It determines the maximum number of shades of gray that can be displayed on the CT monitor, i.e., it determines the range of Hounsfield units represented on a specific image. All values higher than the selected range appear white, and any value lower than the range appears black. Wider windows encompass greater anatomic diversity, but subtle density discrimination is lost. The narrow widths provide greater density discrimination and contrast; and hence it is possible to differentiate the white and gray matter of the brain. Because wider window settings decrease contrast, they suppress the display of noise on an image. For this reason, it is common practice to widen the window when patients are obese or when there are metallic artifacts. **The window level** (WL), on the other hand, is the center or midpoint of the range of CT numbers. The window level should be set at a point that is roughly the same value as the average attenuation number of the tissue of interest. For example WL 50 and WW 200 means that structures having HU values between –50 and 150 are well shown. Some systems provide the option of recording two different window settings, superimposed on one another, in a single image. This technique is known as dual window setting or double window setting. A large window width indicates that there is a relatively long gray scale or a large block of CT numbers that will be assigned some value of gray. Thus, the transition zone between the lower CT numbers portrayed as black and the higher CT numbers portrayed as white will be large. A narrow window width implies that the transition from black to white will take place over a relatively few CT numbers.

Manipulating WW and WL

Wide windows (400 to 2000 HU) should be used trying to encompass tissues of greatly differing attenuation within the image. For example, body scans are usually filmed at 350 to 600 HU to encompass the attenuation numbers of fat, fluid, and muscle. Lung and bone are filmed at 1000 to 2000 to include air spaces and vessels for lung, and cortex and marrow for bone. Narrow windows (50 to 350 HU) should be used to display soft tissues within structures containing different tissues of similar densities. For example, brain may be displayed at 80 to 150 HU to show differences between gray and white matter. Liver may be viewed at 100 to 250 HU to highlight liver metastases. Levels should be centered near the average attenuation of the tissues of interest. For example, body scans may be viewed at about a level of 0 to 60 HU because fat has attenuation numbers from –60 to –100 HU whereas those of muscle and organs may range from about 60 to 150 HU. Lung is viewed at a level of about –600 to –750. Window width has reverse relationship with image contrast.

The WL is the center of the WW. It is the CT number in the middle of the WW and is used to represent the medium gray scale. When the WL is centered on the lungs (lower CT numbers), the image display is optimized for that structure, and the other structures, the liver (soft tissue) and pelvis (bone) are displayed as white. On the other hand, when the WL is centered on the pelvis (higher CT numbers), the image display is optimized for viewing the bony pelvis, and the lungs and liver appear black. Finally, with the WL centered in the middle of the CT number range (in this case, the liver), the pelvis is displayed as white and the liver is optimized for viewing.

IV. PRIORITY RECONSTRUCTION

In new scanners, acquisition speed is substantially faster than image reconstruction speed. This feature may be called priority reconstruction. On demand the last section obtained can be displayed early so that the location of the last section can be confirmed before the patient is shifted from the table.

V. IMAGE MAGNIFICATION

It is important to differentiate between image magnification and decreasing field of view size. A decrease in display field of view increases image size. The result of both functions is an image that appears larger than the original. Image magnification uses only image data, not raw data, and has the effect of stretching the image to a larger size. Magnification does not improve resolution, and image distortion rises with an increase in the magnification factor. But targeted reconstruction using smaller FOV increases the size of the image while increasing the resolution also.

VI. REFERENCE IMAGE

This feature aids in localizing slices according to anatomic landmarks. It is very useful in spine CT to locate the correct vertebral body and also help the neurosurgeon to localize the site of lesion on the table.

VII. SPECIALIZED COMPUTER FOR IMAGE MANIPULATION

There are various other programs available for image manipulation in CT, such as those intended for multiplanar reconstruction, quantitative CT (or osteo-CT), dental CT, 3D imaging, xenon CT, and those that facilitate the use of CT in radiation therapy treatment planning. In addition, there are other programs that provide graphic aids, such as region of interest (ROI), arrows, histogram and annotation.

Multiplanar reconstruction

Multiplanar Reconstruction (MPR) is a computer program intended to create coronal, sagittal and paraxial images from a stack of contiguous transverse axial scans. Whereas the sagittal image defines a plane that passes through an anatomic region from anterior to posterior and divides the body into right and left sections, the coronal image defines a plane that passes through the body region from right to left (or left to right), dividing the region into anterior and posterior sections. The paraxial image, on the other hand, defines a plane that cuts through the coronal and sagittal planes in the longitudinal direction of an anatomic region. Irregular, oblique and other view can also be generated. The irregular view, for example, linear or curved, can be reconstructed from a stack of contiguous transverse images. The oblique views can be reconstructed using at least three arbitrarily definable points in different transverse images. There are several major advantages of reformatted images in CT, including the following:

1. To enable the visualization of specific structure such as the optic nerves and lesions, in relation to surrounding structures.
2. To determine the true extent of lesions or fractures, and to help localize lesions and intra-articular bone fragments or foreign bodies.

One major disadvantage of MPR relates to image quality. Image detail is not as good as that obtained in transaxial images. The reformatted image quality depends on the quality of axial images, and it is therefore important that the patient does not move or breathe during the scanning procedure. In addition, the plane thickness affects image detail, so that thick planes result in blurring and loss of structural detail.

Quantitative CT

Quantitative CT (QCT) or osteo-CT is the most sensitive of all x-ray techniques for measuring the mineral content of trabecular bone in osteoporosis (see Chapter 18).

Histogram

A histogram displays a bar graph to show how frequently a range of CT numbers occurs within an ROI.

Three-dimensional reformation

The individual slices are combined and smoothed so that their merged surfaces resemble the intact patient structure. This feature is called three-dimensional reformation. The most common indications for three-dimensional reformations are trauma, tumor, and birth defects. Three-dimensional image generation often plays a vital role in orthopaedic and reconstructive surgical planning (see Chapter 13).

CHAPTER 7

Radiation Dosimetry

INTRODUCTION

The fascinating developments in CT over the last decade have all tended to increase the number of images obtained during a single CT examination. Because more images can be acquired in an allocated time, and because further data can be obtained with the contrast media techniques, there is a tendency to obtain more and more images during the examination of a single patient. The greater the number of images (particularly through the same anatomical location), the greater will be the radiation dose to key organs such as the ovary and testis. What has been realized only recently is that CT is a major contributor to the medical radiation burden received by the general public. Because of these worries about radiation, it is important that request forms are closely scrutinized to ensure that CT is the most appropriate test and that the required information cannot be obtained by techniques with a lower radiation burden. Of course, these judgments are difficult and are subject to all the deliberations over risk and benefit. Cost and local practicalities come into the equation. Much depends on the relative cost and availability of CT and MRI.

Radiation doses for standard protocols on modern CT system (values in mSv)

	Brain	Chest	Abdomen	L-S-Spine
Orbit	4.8	–	–	–
Parotid	28.8	–	–	–
Thyroid	1.4	3.5	–	–
Lung	–	22.1	15.3	–
Liver	–	4.3	24.1	–
Ovary	–	–	19.4	10.7
Testis	–	–	6.4	1.9
Skin	–	19.0	26.6	–

Estimated effective dose equivalent of common examinations

Examination	Effective dose equivalent
Sinus series, four views	7.0 mrem
Chest, PA and lateral	7.2 mrem
KUB	8.7 mrem
Lumbar spine, five views	125.1 mrem
CT brain	112.0 mrem
CT sinus (160 mAs)	51.2 mrem

Of much more concern is the use of repeated CT examinations for relatively benign disease and the associated cumulative radiation burden. Much of the most worrying area is potential damage to the lens of the eye. Consideration of the use of MRI as an alternative should be given to all requests for CT when repeated studies of benign disease will be required. Likewise, whenever a paediatric patient is referred for CT, the question of whether MRI could be used should be posed. In this regard, it is worth remembering that ultrasound is a very powerful mode of imaging for children. Even when it has been determined that CT is the best test to sort out the clinical problem, it is important to keep the radiation dose down to a minimum (ALARA – as low as reasonably achievable). This can be accomplished by obtaining only those CT images necessary to answer the clinical question. Furthermore, for most thoracic CT, it has now been shown that the mAs can be substantially reduced without compromising image quality. Spiral CT by itself does not increase the radiation dose – assuming comparable factors are used (pitch of 1, volume examined and mAs). However, overlap of exposures (reduced pitch) will lead to increased doses.

FACTORS AFFECTING PATIENT RADIATION DOSE

The ionizing radiation used in CT is the x-ray with maximum kilovoltage of 120 to 140 and average energy near 70 keV. The important factors affecting the radiation dose are

Scanner type (Generation)

The x-ray tube is closer to the patient in a fourth-generation scanner than in a third-generation scanner because it spins inside the detector circle. This proximity increases skin dose slightly.

Rotation angle

Theoretically, a rotation arc of only 180° is required to satisfy most reconstruction algorithms. Most scanners employ 360° acquisition angles to compensate for radiation beam divergence and patient motion. The extra scanning information improves image quality, but increases radiation dose.

Radiographic technique

The tube potential (kilovoltage or kVp) controls the maximum energy of the x-ray beams produced. Typically, scanners operate at 120 to 140 kVp, producing an x-ray spectrum with average photon energy of approximately 70 keV. The kVp setting affects radiographic contrast and dose. As the setting is increased, the radiographic contrast decreases and dose increases if no other changes are made. The ability of the x-ray beam to penetrate tissue also increases, and the ratio of the dose in the center of the slice to the dose at the skin surface increases. The tube current (mA) controls the rate at which x-rays are produced. The scan time controls the duration of exposure. Combined, the mAs controls the total number of x-rays produced. There is a linear relationship between the mAs and the radiation dose. If the mAs is doubled, the total dose doubles.

Filtration

Filtration is required to remove some of the soft, or low energy, x-rays from the beam. The patient would quickly absorb these low-energy x-rays. Photons are needed to penetrate the patient and strike the detectors, but some of them must be absorbed to produce radiographic contrast. Adding metal filters to the beam permits selective removal of x-rays with low energy and reduces the radiation dose while maintaining contrast at an acceptable level. The minimum amount of filtration must be 2.5 mm of aluminium-equivalent material for machines that operate above 90 kVp.

Collimation

Leaded collimators are used near the x-ray tube to control the size of the beam striking the patient. If the radiation beam were not controlled to match the detector size, then there would be additional scatter radiation to degrade the image and produce excessive radiation dose to the patient.

Detector efficiency

Solid-state detectors typically have high efficiency (90%-100%) and require the least amount of radiation exposure. These detectors are commonly used in third and fourth-generation scanners. Pressurized gas detectors, such as xenon, typically are less efficient (50%-60%) and require more radiation dose for the same image statistics.

Scan field diameter

If the displayed field is smaller than the scanned field, the area outside the displayed field of view is still irradiated, but with no image information. Larger fields irradiate more tissue and allow more potential scatter to degrade the image. However, for the same radiographic technique (kVp and mAs), a smaller scan field often produces higher radiation doses than a large field because of the greater concentration of radiation from the rotation of the x-ray beam focused on a smaller volume of tissue. Absorbed dose is volume dependent.

Slice thickness and spacing

As slice thickness increases, the volume of tissue irradiated increases and the dose may increase slightly in the slice. However, for multiple-slice examinations, decreasing slice thickness and using contiguous slices will increase the MSAD because of the increased amount of scatter radiation to adjacent slices. Also, to maintain image quality (noise) at the same level, additional radiation is needed for thinner slices.

Patient size

Large patients or thick body parts often require radiographic techniques that increase the radiation dose.

Repeat scans

Areas of the patient that are rescanned for contrast studies or other technical or clinical reasons receive additional radiation. The effect is cumulative.

Image matrix size

Increasing the matrix size from 512 to 1024 quadruples the number of pixels in the matrix increases the spatial resolution capabilities, but requires additional radiation dose to maintain the same statistics in each pixel.

Spiral technique

With a spiral technique and a pitch of 1:1, there is no difference in radiation dose relative to axial techniques.

Localization scans (Scanogram)

The radiation dose for these scanned slit projection radiography techniques is low, on the order of 25 to 100 mrad.

Reconstruction filters

Reconstruction filters do not affect the radiation dose to the patient unless they change the radiographic technique.

CHAPTER

8

CT Image Quality

1. INTRODUCTION

In conventional radiography, essentially there are five characteristics of the radiographic image that determine its quality–spatial resolution, contrast resolution, noise, distortion and artifacts. Each of these is influenced by a number of factors related to processing, geometry, motion, subject contrast, film contrast technique, image receptor, focal spot size, viewing conditions and observer performance. Essentially, image quality in CT depends on spatial resolution, contrast resolution, noise and artifacts. Even though image quality is subjective in many aspects, the major factors, spatial and density resolution, can be quantitatively specified.

2. SPATIAL RESOLUTION

Spatial resolution is defined as the ability to present small objects and differentiate between closely spaced objects. Spatial resolution is used to describe the degree of blurring present in an image. For a CT scanner, spatial resolution "is a measure of the ability to discriminate object of varying density a small distance apart against a uniform background". It is a measure of the accuracy in depicting anatomical structures. It is most commonly described in terms of the Full Width Half Maximum (FWHM). This parameter is the measure of how well a point is reproduced in the image. The FWHM is the width of the curve at the point where the attenuation values are 50% of peak value. The smaller the width (i.e. FWHM) better the resolution. Another method of examining spatial resolution is to consider line images. This ability to distinguish separate lines in an image would measure spatial resolution. It can be stated in terms of number of lines per centimeter that can be visualized in the image. The spatial resolution is affected by many design parameters. They are

I. Choice of filter
II. Geometric factors
   1. Size of detector aperture
   2. Focal spot size and milliampere settings
   3. Slice thickness
   4. Focus to isocenter and focus to detector distance
III. No. of projection profiles obtained
IV. Matrix (pixel) size
V. Contrast
VI. Reconstruction algorithm

Effect of filters

For a crisp image high spatial frequencies are accentuated. This causes sharpening of edges and improved resolution. Noise increase and the density resolution diminish with accentuation of high spatial frequency.

Geometric factors

Geometric factors refer to factors that play a role in the data acquisition process. These include the focal spot size, detector aperture width, slice thickness, the focus to isocenter and focus to detector distance.

Use of a small filament size concentrates the focal spot and improves spatial resolution. Unfortunately, small filaments cannot tolerate a high level of milliamperes. Therefore, systems that offer higher milliampere settings usually provide two separate filaments. A small filament is provided for lower milliampere settings and a large filament for higher settings. In reality, the loss of resolution caused by a larger filament is slight, and it is nearly impossible to see on a standard CT image. If too low a milliampere-second setting is used, the image does not appear too light, as would a chest x-ray, rather, the underexposed CT image has a grainy appearance because an insufficient number of x-ray photons reach the detectors. An overexposed CT image is not seriously degraded, although some streaking artifacts are possible. In CT, the effective focal spot size at the isocenter represents the size of the focal spot in the x-ray tube. If the effective focal spot size increases, details in the object are distributed over several detectors, thus decreasing the spatial resolution.

The aperture size refers to the width of the aperture at the detector. Generally, when the aperture size is smaller than the spacing between objects, the objects can be resolved. This means that for smaller aperture sizes, higher spatial resolution can be obtained. Both the focal spot size and detector aperture width affect resolution in terms of the effective scan beam width at the isocenter. The focus-to-isocenter and focus-to-detector distances affect beam width. Smaller focal spots and smaller detector aperture widths improve spatial resolution. Imaging small objects faithfully, that is, with excellent spatial resolution depends on the slice thickness, or collimation. For example, if the object size is 4 mm, a 10 mm slice thickness results in spreading the 4 mm object over the entire slice thickness, and the result would be an incorrect CT number. This effect is called the partial volume effect. A slice thickness close to the object size – say, 5 mm slice thickness – would be a significant improvement, thus increasing spatial resolution. Resolution could be increased without limit by reducing the aperture opening but limitations are cost of manufacture and increase in radiation dose as the number of photons reaching the detector decrease (to compensate).

Number of projection profiles

Another factor influencing spatial resolution is the number of projections. As the number of projections increases, more data are available for image reconstruction and better spatial resolution results. To obtain resolution of 1 mm with small or average-sized bodies 700-800 views may be needed. In many machines those needs are exceeded significantly allowing spatial resolution down to 0.5 mm range.

Matrix size

The spatial resolution can be better than the size represented by the pixel length. In reality the pixel size should be 1.5-2 times smaller than the desired resolution. It must be realized that the pixel size refers to the field or body not the viewing screen or film.

Reconstruction algorithm

The next category of factors affecting spatial resolution is the reconstruction algorithm. Essentially, if the projection profiles are back-projected without correction, then blurring results. To sharpen the image, a convolution process, basically a high-pass filter, is applied to weight the scan profiles prior to back-projection. The convolution algorithm affects the appearance of image structures. In general, these algorithms are applied to emphasize soft tissue and bone and are known as the soft tissue and bone detail algorithms. Whereas the former is applied to the pancreas, adrenal, lung nodules, or any soft tissue region, the latter, the bone algorithm, is applied to bony structures, such as the inner ear and dense bone. Spatial resolution at high contrast is also called high-contrast resolution. Display resolution in CT is defined as the number of pixels per horizontal and vertical dimensions of the matrix on the monitor screen or film sheet. Today CT scanners use higher matrix sizes in conjunction with selected convolution algorithms to improve display resolution.

3. DENSITY RESOLUTION (CONTRAST RESOLUTION)

It is the ability to differentiate the attenuation coefficient of adjacent pieces of tissue. In the computation of any one pixel value there is error in the form of statistical variation and it is this variation which limits the ultimate density resolution. This variation is called as image noise and manifest as grainy background or mottle. The parameter used to evaluate this variation is standard deviation.

For example, standard deviation equal to 5 HU on a Hounsfield scale of ($\pm$) 1000 would translate to 5 HU | 1000 HU = 0.5%. The interpretation is that two adjacent pixels are not significantly different if their CT numbers vary by less than or equal to 5 HU. Noise is the ultimate limitation in the accuracy of density resolution. Parameters that affect or induce noise need to be understood.

1) Scan Geometry
2) X-ray scatter
3) Computation-induced error
4) Frequency response
5) Voxel size

Scan geometry

Although a 360^0 tube rotation per scan is the most common selection, it is not the only choice. It is possible to obtain a partial scan, which is acquired from 180^0 plus the degree of arc of the fan angle. Although this scan is slightly more than a half circle, these scans are often referred to as half-scans. Only half of the data are available to reconstruct the image with partial scan; therefore, they are inferior to standard 360^0 scan. Another tube arc option is the 400^0 scan, known as an overscan. The overscan adds approximately the width of the field of view to a full scan. These are more commonly used in fourth-generation scanner designs.

Scanning parameters

Many scanning parameters affect the quality of the image produced. Some of these variables can be regulated by the operator, whereas others, such as patient size, cannot. Among the factors that the operator can control are millampere (mA) level, scan time, slice thickness, field of view, and scan algorithm. On some systems, the operator may adjust the kilovolt-peak (kVp) setting, although on many systems, it is fixed at 120 kVp. Large photon flux reduces noise but increases the radiation dose level. The patient and presence of high attenuating materials affect detected intensity and in turn the uncertainty in measurement. A large patient will have more mottled image. Similarly presence of high contrast objects causes increased noise.

X-ray scatter

The amount of scattering that is detected is controlled by collimation of the detectors. Small aperture reduces scattering. Scanners using wide aperture have greater noise.

Voxel size

The measured intensity is also affected by the voxel length i.e. if slice thickness is reduced to 50% the detector, collimator size must also be reduced accordingly which reduces the intensity by the same amount. To retain the same accuracy requires restoration of the detected photon intensity, which means doubling the dose. Similarly decreasing pixel size increases the relative inaccuracy unless the photon flux is raised. Basically density resolution is related to spatial resolution and these two factors of image quality cannot be treated completely separately.

QUALITY CONTROL

Quality control has become common in radiology departments and is now an integral part of equipment testing and maintenance programs in hospitals. Quality control ensures that the CT scanner is performing optimally through a series of tests that are conducted daily, monthly, and annually. These tests include those for spatial resolution, contrast resolution, noise, slice width, kVp waveform, average CT number of water, standard deviation of CT numbers in water, radiation scatter and leakage, and a host of others, which constitute a generic quality control program for CT scanners.

CHAPTER

9

CT Image Artifacts

An artifact is "a distortion or error in an image that is unrelated to the subject being studied." In addition to noise, artifacts can degrade image quality and affect the perceptibility of detail.

Motion

Voluntary and involuntary motion of the patient during CT scanning result in the appearance of streak artifacts on the image, which appear tangential to high-contrast edges of the moving part. These streaks appear because it is difficult for the algorithm to deal with inconsistencies in the voxel attenuation arising from the edge of the moving part.

Metal

The presence of metal in the patient also causes artifacts. Metallic materials such as prosthetic devices, dental fillings, surgical clips, and electrodes give rise to streak artifacts on the image. Metal artifacts can be reduced by using an appropriate computer program, such as the Metal Artifact Reduction (MAR) program described by Felsenberg and associates.

Beam hardening

Beam hardening refers to the increase in the mean energy of a polychromatic beam (the x-ray beam in CT) as it passes through an object (patient). Lower energy photons are absorbed as the beam passes through the object. Because of this, the CT numbers of certain structures change. This change in CT numbers results in beam hardening artifacts, which appear as broad dark bands or streaks. This is known as the "cupping" artifact. It can be seen when scanning the brain, and appears as "an increase in CT numbers for the soft tissue along the bone-tissue transition of the vault of the cranium and posterior fossa." These CT numbers decrease toward the middle of the CT section, hence the term "cupping". Beam hardening artifacts can be reduced or eliminated by the use of beam hardening correction programs.

Partial volume effect

When CT numbers are computed, the calculations are based on the linear attenuation coefficients for a voxel of tissue. If the voxel contains only one tissue type, then there is no problem with the calculation. For example, if the tissue in the voxel is dense bone, the CT number is computed to be 1000. On the other hand, if the voxel now contains three similar tissue types in which the CT numbers are close together – for example, blood (CT number = 40), gray matter (CT number = 43), and white matter (CT number = 46) then the CT number for that voxel is based on an average of the three tissues (i.e. the CT number is 43). This is known as partial volume averaging. Partial volume averaging can give rise to the partial volume effect which leads to partial volume artifacts. By scanning thinner slices, the partial volume artifact can be minimized. Another method that can be used to reduce partial volume artifacts is a computerised technique called the Volume Artifact Reduction (VAR) technique.

Ring artifacts

An artifact characteristic of third-generation CT scanners is the ring artifact, which arises as a result of one or more bad detectors. The reason for the ring is that during the rotation of the x-ray tube and detector array, the rays measured by a given detector are tangent to a circle. If a detector has an offset or gain difference of 0.1% with neighbouring detectors, a circular artifact will be present in the image. Such an artifact indicates that the detector gain needs to be calibrated. A faulty detector in a fourth-generation scanner does not give rise to a noticeable artifact because each detector acquires a view and the bad data are spread evenly across the image. Also, detector-to-detector channel variations rarely create a problem in a fourth-generation scanner because the detector is calibrated by the raw radiation beam during a scan.

Troubleshooting in artifacts on the CT image

Artifact	Problem	Rectification
1. Ring	Detector problem: more common on third-generation scanners because the tube and detector move together, rarely seen on fourth generations	Recalibrate: If rings persist, call service

(Contd.)

Artifact	Problem	Rectification
2. Aliasing effect	Too few samples	If partial scan was used, rescan with a complete arc; increase scan time.
3. Edge gradient effect (straight line radiating from high-con trast areas, such as bone or soft tissue.)	Angle of x-ray beam varies between two similar views.	Increase scan time, decrease slice thickness
4. Beam hardening artifact–broad streaks, cupping (periphery of image is lighter), vague areas of low density	X-ray beams are composed of different energies	Increase kilovolt-peak setting; decrease slice thickness; decrease milli-ampere level, increase filtration
5. Noise (grainy appearance)	Insufficient photons reaching detectors, may be caused by low milliampere level, low tube output	Increase milliampere level; increase slice thickness; call service
6. Out-of-field artifact (shading at the periphery of the image)	Patient is not entirely enclosed in scan field	Increase scan field size
7. Air-contrast interface artifact	Significant difference in density between contrast and air; motion may contribute; most frequent in gastric air-fluid level.	Rescan patient in a decubitus or prone position if necessary
8. Lines on scout image	Faulty detector	Call service

CHAPTER 10

Components and Equipment Specifications of a CT Scanner

INTRODUCTION

The major systems of a CT scanner include :

1) The imaging system
2) Computer system
3) Image display, recording and storage system.

The three major systems are housed in three separate rooms: The imaging system is located in the scanner room. The computer system is in the com-

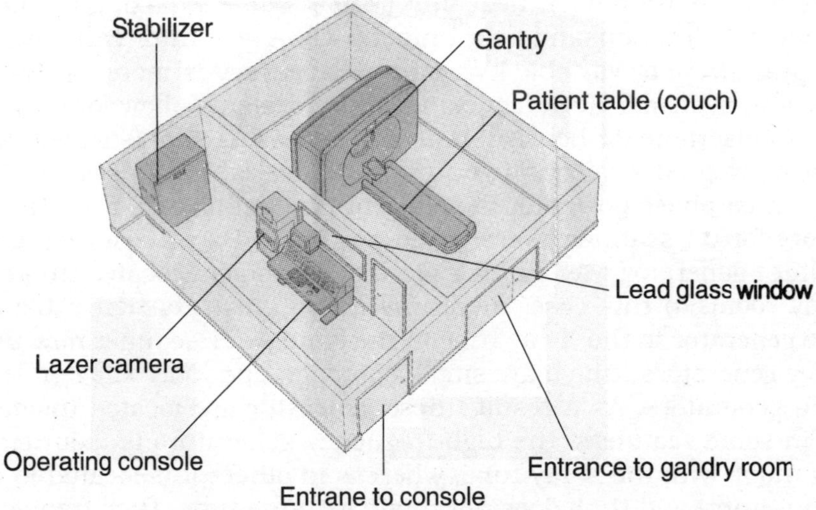

Fig 10.1. Aerial view of CT scan room.

puter room. The display, recording, and storage system is located in the operator's room.

IMAGING SYSTEM

The imaging system is composed of several components working together to acquire an image from the patient and are housed in the gantry. The gantry and patient couch are often referred to as the scanner. The major components of imaging system are generator, collimators, filter, detectors and detector electronics. The X-ray tube and generator are responsible for X-ray production. The radiation beam emerging from the tube is filtered through a specially designed filter that not only protects the patient from low-energy rays but also ensures that a more uniform beam falls on the detectors. The collimators in the CT help to define the slice thickness and restrict the X-ray beam only to the cross section of interest. Finally, while the detectors capture the X-ray photons and convert them into electrical signals (analog information), the detector electronics - the data acquisition system (DAS), as it is often referred to-converts this information into digital data.

A. X-RAY SYSTEM

The components of the X-ray system include the X-ray generator, X-ray tube, the X-ray beam filter, and collimator.

X-ray generator

The generator produces high voltage and transmits it to the X-ray tube. The power capacity of the generator is listed in kilowatts (kW). Also listed the anode heat capacity (in million heat unit (MHU) and the maximum anode heat dissipation rate (in thousand heat units (kHU). A generator can have a single kilovolt-peak (kVp) or variable kVp output. Accuracy is more easily achieved in single kVp systems. However, variable kVp systems allow for an increased capacity to discriminate between different tissues. A sophisticated generator is necessary to produce accurate output with a variable kVp system. CT scanners use three-phase power for the efficient production of X-rays. In the past, generators for CT scanners were based on the 60 Hz voltage frequency, and high voltage generator was a bulky piece of equipment located in a corner of the X-ray room. In this case, there was a long, high-tension cable running from the generator to the X-ray tube in the gantry. CT scanner now uses high frequency generators, which are small, compact, and more efficient than conventional generators. As a result, these generator are located inside the CT gantry. In some scanners, the high frequency generators is mounted on the rotating frame with the X-ray tube, whereas in others it is located in one corner of the gantry and thus does not rotate with the tube. High frequency generators are based on higher frequencies than the 60 Hz supplies. In this situation, the 60 Hz is converted to 400–2000 Hz and after rectification and smoothing the ripple from these generators is less than 1% compared to 4% from three-phase, 12 pulse, conventional generates. This makes the high frequency generator more efficient at X-ray production than its previous counterpart.

Filtration

Radiation from X-ray tube is polychromatic consisting of long and short wave length. One assumption in clinical CT is that the beam is monochromatic, but it is actually polychromatic. It is essential, therefore, that the polychromatic beam be shaped so that it appears to be a monochromatic beam to satisfy the requirements of the reconstruction process. This requires the use of a special filter. In CT, filtration serves a dual purpose. It removes long wavelength X-rays, because they do not play a role in CT image formation but contribute to patient dose. The result of filtration is that the mean energy of the beam increases and the beam becomes "harder". This can give rise to beam hardening artifacts. It also shapes the energy distribution across the radiation beam to produce uniform beam hardening when X-rays pass through the filter and the object. Filtering the X-ray beam with a substance such as Teflon or aluminium helps to reduce the range of X-ray energies that reach the patient. Creating a more uniform beam intensity improves the CT image by reducing artifacts. These mechanical filters shape the X-ray beam intensity. Filtering removes soft or low-energy, X-ray beams and minimizes patient exposure. Certain filters are used to reduce the beam intensity at the periphery of the beam, corresponding to the thinner areas of patient's anatomy. Filtering produces a smaller degree of photon intensity. Because of their shape, they are often referred to as bow tie filters. There are also software corrections that can be made after the X-ray beams are attenuated by the patient, reducing the effect of beam hardening of the image.

The X-ray tube

The heat storage capacity and cooling rates of the tube are especially important. With respect to detectors, the type, quantum detection, and conversion efficiencies are also important. Formerly, first- and second-generation scanners used fixed anode, oil-cooled X-ray tubes but, because of the demand for increasing output resulting from faster scan times typical of modern CT scanners, rotating anode X-ray tubes have become common in CT. These tubes produce the heterogeneous beam of radiation from a large diameter anode disk with focal spot sizes to facilitate the spatial resolution requirements of the scanner. The disk is usually made of rhenium, tungsten and molybdenum alloy with small target angle and a rotation speed of 3600 rpm. The focal spot size varies. Dual focal spot system with 0.6 × 1.6 mm for the small and 0.9 × 2.4 mm for the large is an example. The introduction of spiral CT made possible with continuous rotation scanners has placed new demand on X-ray tubes. Because of the continuous rotation of the tube for a longer period of time, it must be capable of sustaining higher power levels. One significant change in X-ray tubes for slip ring scanners is that they are designed to increase not only the heat storage capacity but also the cooling rate (heat dissipation).

Collimation

In CT, collimation is important because it affects not only patient dose but also image quality. Two types are clearly apparent – pre-patient collimators and post-patient collimators. It is important to note that these detectors must be in perfect alignment to optimize the imaging process. In general, a set of collimator sections is carefully arranged to shape the beam, which is proximal to the focal spot. The collimators, both proximal and distal, are arranged to ensure the constant beam width at the detector. Detector collimators also shape the beam and help remove scattered radiation. The collimator section at the distal end of the collimator assembly also helps the defined thickness of the slice to be imaged.

B. SCANNING GANTRY

The gantry is a framework mounted so that it surrounds the patients in a vertical plane. It contains the rotating scan frame on to which is mounted the X-ray generator and X-ray tube. The gantry also houses other imaging components such as the slip rings, collimators, detectors and detector electronics. The generator in the gantry is usually a small, solid state, high frequency generator mounted on the rotating scan frames and operating at about 5-50 kHz. It is located close to the X-ray tube so that only a short length of high-tension cable is required to couple the X-ray tube and generator. During operation of the scanner, the X-ray tube produces heat. With numerous components in the gantry, of which several are affected by the ambient air temperature gantry cooling is of prime consideration. The gantry aperture refers to the opening in which the patient is positioned during the scanning procedure. The aperture is such that the technologist can approach the patient from the front and back of the gantry. Most scanners have a 70 cm aperture, a size that facilitates positioning the patient and helps provide access to patients in emergency situations. X-ray energy is emitted as the tube travels along this path to reach the patient, who is placed within the opening. Some of the X-ray energy passes through the patient, and some is attenuated or scattered. The X-ray beams that pass through the patient are retrieved by the computer detectors.

C. PATIENT COUCH

The patient's couch or patient table provides a platform on which the patient lies during the CT examination. The couch consists of a support referred to as a couch top, which rests on a pedestal. The couch top is usually made of

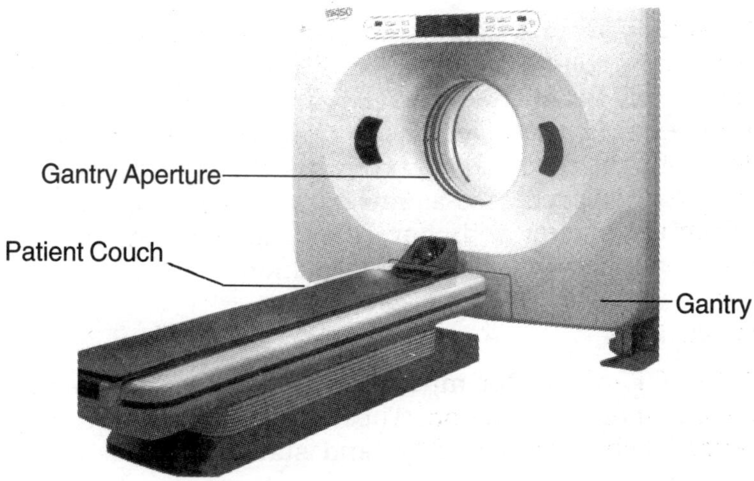

Fig. 10.2. CT Scanner

carbon fiber composites, because they have low absorption and excellent vibration damping features and meets the strength requirements necessary for imaging heavy patient. Two couch movements vital to any CT examination are those in the vertical and horizontal directions. The vertical movement should provide a range of height from the floor to make it easy for patients to get on and off the table. Horizontal or longitudinal couch movements should enable the patient to be scanned from head to thighs without the need for repositioning. particularly the movement characteristics and strength of the couch top. The process of moving the table by a specified measure is most commonly called incrementation, but is also referred to as feed, step or index.

D. CT DETECTOR SYSTEM

Detectors currently in use are made of either xenon gas or solid-state crystals. Pressurized xenon gas fills hollow chambers to produce detectors that absorb approximately 60% to 87% of the photons that reach them. Xenon gas detectors are significantly less expensive to produce, somewhat easier to calibrate and highly stable. A xenon detector channel consists of three tungsten plates. When a photon enters the channel, it ionizes the xenon gas. These ions are accelerated and amplified by the electric field between the plates. The collected charge produces an electric current. This current is then processed as raw data. A disadvantage of xenon gas is that it must be kept under pressure in an aluminium casing. Solid-state crystal detectors are made from a variety of materials, including sodium iodide, bismuth germinate, cadmium tungstate, cesium iodide, and ceramic rare earth. They absorb nearly 100% of photons that reach them. In addition, there is no loss in the front window, as in xenon systems. This increased absorption efficiency is the chief advantage of solid-state detectors. Solid-state detectors may produce a brief afterglow. However, new solid-state detectors reduce or eliminate this disadvantage. When an X-ray beam strikes a solid-state detector, it is absorbed by the scintillator material in the detector. This material then generates a corresponding level of light. The detector converts the light levels into an electric current, which is then processed as raw data. CT detectors capture the radiation beam from the patient and convert it in to electrical signals, which are subsequently converted into digital information.

Detector characteristics

To be useful in CT, a detector must exhibit several characteristics that are essential for CT image production. These include efficiency, response time, dynamic range, high reproducibility, and stability. Efficiency refers to the ability to capture, absorb, and convert X-ray photons to electrical signals. CT detectors must possess high capture efficiency, high absorption efficiency, and high conversion efficiency. Capture efficiency refers to the efficiency with which the detectors can obtain photons transmitted from the patient. Absorption efficiency refers to the number of photons absorbed by the detector, and this depends on the atomic number, physical density, size, and thickness of the detector face. Stability refers to the steadiness of the detector response. If the system is not stable, frequent calibrations are required to render the signals useful. The response time of the detector refers to the speed with which the detector can detect an X-ray event and recover to detect another event. Response times should be very short to avoid problems such as afterglow and detector "pile-up". Finally, the dynamic range of a CT detector is the "ratio of the largest signal to be measured to the precision of the smallest signal to be discriminated".

Characteristics of detectors

Solid-state crystal	*Pressurized xenon gas*
High photon absorption	Moderate photon absorption
Sensitive to temperature moisture	Highly stable
Solid material	Low-density material (gas)
Can exhibit afterglow	No afterglow
No front window loss	Losses due to front window and the spaces taken by plates

The conversion of X-rays to electrical energy in a detector is based on two fundamental principles. Some detectors convert X-ray energy first into light, and then the light is converted into electrical energy; these are called scintillation detectors. Other detectors convert X-ray energy directly to electrical energy; these are referred to as gas ionization detectors.

Scintillation detectors

Scintillation detectors consist of a scintillation crystal coupled to a photomultiplier tube. When X-rays fall on to the crystal, flashes of light (scintillations) are produced. The light is then directed to the photomultiplier (PM) tube. The light from the crystal strikes the photocathode of the PM tube, which releases electrons. These electrons, in turn, cascade through a series of diodes, carefully arranged in the tube and maintained at different potentials, which give rise to a small output signal. In the past, early scanners used sodium iodide (NaI) crystals coupled to PM tubes. Later, because of afterglow problems and the limited dynamic range of NaI, other crystals such as calcium fluoride and bismuth germinate were used. Today, scintillation detectors with PM tubes have been superseded by solid-state photodiode multiplier scintillation crystal detectors. Two scintillation materials that are currently used with photodiodes are cadmium tungstate ($CdWO_4$) and a ceramic material made of high purity, rare earth oxides.

Gas ionization detectors

The other type of CT detector is based on the principle of ionization. These gas ionization detectors were introduced with the development of third-generation scanners. It consists of a series of individual gas chambers usually separated by tungsten plates carefully positioned so that they act as electron collection plates. When X-rays fall on the individual cells (ionization of the gas) it results in producing positive and negative ions. The positive ions migrate to the negatively charged plate, whereas the negative ions are attracted to the positively charged plate. This migration of ions gives rise to a small signal current that varies directly with the number of photons absorbed.

Detector electronics : Data acquisition system

The Data Acquisition System (DAS) refers to the detector electronics positioned between the detector array and computer. Because the DAS is located between the detectors and the computer, it plays the role of a translator by performing three major functions :

1. Measuring the transmitted radiation beam;
2. Encoding these measurements in to binary data; and
3. Transmit the binary or digital data in to the computer.

The components of the DAS are intended to handle these functions. The detector measures the transmitted X-rays from the patient and converts them into electrical energy. This electrical signal is so weak that it must be amplified before it can be analyzed further, the preamplifier does this. Another function of the DAS is logarithmic conversion- that is, the transmission measurement data must be changed into attenuation and thickness data.

COMPUTER SYSTEM

The computer system receives the digital data from the DAS of the imaging system and processes it to reconstruct an image of the cross-sectional anatomy. In addition, the computer system performs image manipulation and wide variety of image processing operations, ranging from windowing, image enhancement, image enlargement, measurements, multiplanar reconstruction to three-dimensional imaging and quantitative measurements. The computer system generally includes input-output devices, central processing units, array processors, interface devices, back projector processor, storage devices, and communications hardware. The computer system also includes the software, which enables each hardware component to perform specific tasks.

Computer and image processing system

The computer and image processing system consist of mainly three elements—processing architecture, hardware and software. Currently, computer architecture in CT is capable of multiprocessing, a mode of operation in which two or more connected and roughly equal processing units each carry out one or more processes in tandem. These architectures facilitate parallel processing, distributed processing or pipeline processing.

Pipeline processing

This architecture allows for extremely rapid image reconstruction so that after scanning is completed the image can be viewed on the monitor. Pipeline processing enables the significant reconstruction steps of preprocessing convolution and back projection to be assigned to separate processors.

Parallel processing

A parallel processing architecture is called parallax. The architecture consists of three multitask computers coupled by means of the system bus and distributed among the scan, display, and file processors.

Distributed processing

An example of distributed processing is the back-projector processor which is characterized by its multiple pipeline architecture and therefore passes views sequentially at pipeline speeds of 80 nsec/pixel. There are two other processor boards, one for the digital laser camera and the other specifically intended for the monitor and keyboard. Finally, there is a CPU board coupled to the CT console and storage devices.

CT software

The software for CT includes modules for the following :

1. ***Operator communications*** : The operator must be able to communicate with the system to enable scanning, which may be activated through the use of keyboard commands or by a touch screen.
2. Control of the scanner and image reconstruction
3. ***Image display and manipulation*** : There is a wide range of image display and manipulation techniques afforded by the CT software.
4. ***Operating systems*** : These are programs that control the hardware components of the computer, so they control its overall operation and enable it to run other programs as well. The operating system consists of a major program called the supervisor, which resides in primary memory and controls all other portions of the operating system. CT computers, by virtue of their operating systems, often take advantage of what has been referred to as interleaved processing techniques, such as multitasking, multiprocessing, and multiprogramming. These techniques allow computers to process several programs almost simultaneously, thus increasing the number of jobs the computer can handle in any given time. In addition, the system runs rapidly and efficiently. The operating system used in some CT systems is a UNIX-compatible operating system that facilitates multiuser and multitasking capabilities.

IMAGE DISPLAY, RECORD AND STORAGE SYSTEM

Processed CT images (digital images) can be stored for later retrieval, displayed for immediate viewing, and recorded permanently on to X-ray film. The purpose of image display, record and storage (IDRS) system is threefold:

1. To display the output digital image from the computer in a form meaningful to the observer.
2. To provide a hardcopy of the image on a recording medium.
3. To facilitate the storage and retrieval of vast amount of the digital data. Currently, CT images are displayed on cathode ray tubes (CRT's) recorded on X-ray film, and stored on magnetic tapes and disks and/or optical disks.

Image display

The operator prior to recording and storing the final image displays CT images on a monitor for viewing and manipulation. In general, a display device for CT is a black and white or colour monitor (cathode ray tube, CRT). Whereas images are usually displayed in gray scale, non-image data such as text fields, patient data, and option selection can be displayed in colour. Now-a-days interactive coloring is available for three-dimensional images also. A gray scale monitor is a CRT display device that is funnel-shaped, evacuated glass envelope with an electron gun at the narrow end of the tube. The expanded end of the tube forms a screen, the inner surface of which is coated with a phosphor that emits light when struck by electrons. In CT, the digital image from the computer must be converted into analog signals by the digital-to-analog converter. These signals produce an electron beam that scans the phosphor screen. The scanning is such that the gray scale monitor can display the input digital image pixel by pixel. One important physical parameter of the gray scale display monitor is resolution. It is related to the size of the pixel matrix (matrix size).

IMAGE STORAGE

Because CT is a digital imaging modality, data are stored in digital form to preserve the wide dynamic range of images, including the capability for image processing and intensity transformations, and to decrease the possibility of lost records and reduce the space needed for archiving. Digital images are stored in two-dimensional pixel arrays, with each pixel points represented by a number of bits that determine how many gray levels can be represented by a particular pixel. A typical CT image has a matrix size of 512 × 512 × 8 to 12 bits deep. A CT image of 512 × 512 × 2 bytes (16 bits) deep would require 0.5 MB of storage. If the CT examination contains about 50 images, then the total storage needed is 25 MB. If 50 examinations are done in any one day, 1.25 GB of storage are needed. Storage devices for CT include magnetic tape and disks, digital videotape, optical disks, and optical tapes.

Hard copy recording : The laser recording system

The requirements for hard copy recording (film recording) of CT images are stringent, because these images are used for diagnostic interpretation. The requirements are broad gray scale contrast resolution and high spatial resolution to enable subtle differences in tissue contrast to be perceived and to detect boundaries of different tissues, respectively. These requirements are met by two types of film recording systems—multiformat video camera recording and laser electronic image recording. Whereas multiformat video cameras were popular in the past, laser cameras are now in common use. A laser image recording system, or laser printer, is expensive and sophisticated piece of electronic equipment. It consists of several major components, of which the laser and recording material are important to the CT technologist. This is because the film must match the spectral emission (wavelength) of the laser light. Two types of lasers are available for film recording in CT, solid-state laser diodes and gas lasers, such as helium-neon (He-Ne), helium-cadmium, argon, carbon dioxide, and nitrogen. Of the gas lasers, the helium-neon is the simplest and very reliable. The steps in printing a film using a laser printer can be summarised as follows. On receiving the appropriate command from the operator, the unexposed film is transported to the exposure region of the printer. Once in the exposure region, the film is scanned systematically, line by line, whereby the laser receives its signal from the computer to produce a latent image. Depending on the printer, the laser-scanned film is sent to a receiving magazine (or to a chemical processor coupled to the printer), where it is developed. The result is a laser-printed film ready for viewing.

OPERATOR'S CONSOLE

CT control consoles have evolved into what have come to be known as the integrated type, as well as the type based on the multimedia concept. In general, an integrated console consists of a floating keyboard, an operating panel, a floppy disk drive, and a video display monitor. The integrated console controls the entire system, including turning the scanner on and off, and also enables a number of different functions to be carried out. It is worthwhile to consider the characteristics of the display monitor and keyboard and of the touch panel control. The general ergonomics should be considered as well (the term "ergonomics" refers to the study of how people interact with the equipment in their working environment; it addresses issues relating to comfort, efficiency, and safety in the design of the equipment and the environment). Film recording and storage considerations should also be addressed. A major control console device is the floating keyboard, which can be conveniently positioned to facilitate ease of use. Depending on the keyboard, several controls are prominent and important to the CT technologist. This includes alpha numeric and special function keys, the tract ball or mouse, and window controls. The purpose of a touch panel (it is the screen that the operator is touching) is to allow for system parameters, such as scan setup and control parameters, to be actuated without the need for typing commands at the keyboard. Window controls include the window width and window level controls, which are used to alter picture contrast. CT control consoles usually feature floppy disk drives.

OPTIONS AND ACCESSORIES FOR CT SYSTEM

CT vendors provide a wide variety of hardware and software options and accessories for their CT imaging system. CT hardware options range from optical disks, remote diagnostic stations to independent workstations, multiformat video cameras, and laser cameras. Software options include packages for bone mineral analysis, dynamic scan, 3D image reconstruction, virtual endoscopy, volumetric multiplanar reformatting, evaluation of regional cerebral blood flow (xenon CT), dental CT, and networking. Accessories for CT scanners are

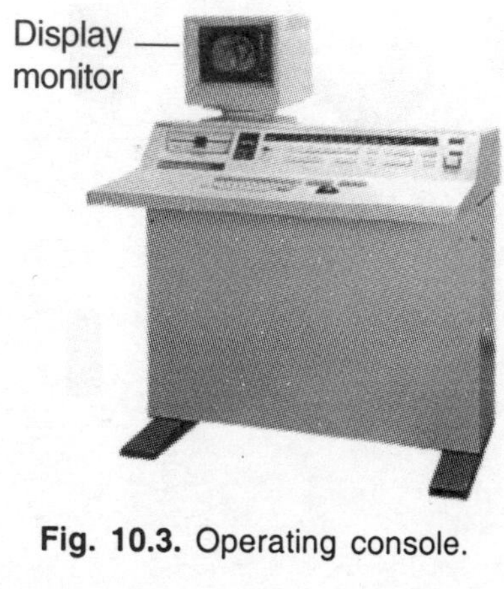

Fig. 10.3. Operating console.

devices that support and provide excellent immobilization of the patient during the scanning procedure to enhance the overall efficiency of the CT examination. These accessories include a pediatric cradle, arm and leg support, table mattress, side rails, table extender, knee support, head pillow with hand rests, axial and coronal head holders, and autotraction straps.

ROOM LAYOUT FOR CT EQUIPMENT

The room layout for CT scanners varies among institutions and depends on the particular type of scanner. In general, a typical room layout includes at least two sections or rooms to house different components of the scanner: The scanning room houses the gantry and patient couch. This room should be large enough to accommodate stretchers (trolleys) and emergency equipment. Directorate of radiation safety recommends minimum space of 25 squire metres with minimum 4 metres breadth for the scanning room. The control room houses the control console and film recording equipment.

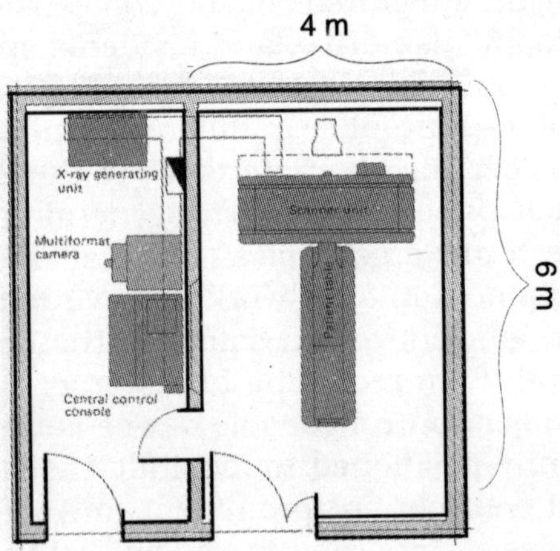

Fig. 10.4. Typical room layout for a CT scanner.

CHAPTER 11

Introduction to Routine Scan Procedures

INTRODUCTION

Ideally all CT examinations should be a tailor-made examination rather than a protocol-based investigation. The aim of the study should be to solve a particular problem without subjecting the patient to unnecessary radiation and keeping his expenses to the minimum. If a doubt can be cleared by two sections, only two sections are enough instead of an elaborate study according to the general protocol. However many protocols have been evolved over a period for most of the CT examinations. These protocols are very useful to the beginners; at the same time these will provide uniformity of the examination at least in majority of the studies worldwide so that comparison between studies done at two different centers is easy. I do suggest the beginners to follow some standard protocols until they are habituated with exactly what a clinician require from a radiologist and the patient actually needs. In general the protocols of Conentional CT (CCT) and spiral CT can be discussed under the following headings.

INDICATIONS

It is must for the technologist to know the indications for a CT examination. As soon as he receives the request form should go through the details regarding the area to be scanned, request for particular method of scanning, regarding use of contrast media etc thoroughly. Sometimes in a particular case routine protocols may not be suitable.

3. PATIENT HISTORY

It is important to include in the patient's history any previous medical conditions and surgeries as well as current symptoms. It is also helpful to record when the symptoms began and whether the condition is new or chronic. Because scarring caused by radiation therapy often mimics lung disease, it is important to note previous oncology treatments.

ENHANCEMENT TECHNIQUES

All CT systems allow a notation concerning contrast media. Often, the notation +C is added for studies after the introduction of contrast medium. Routine procedure for many CT examinations includes scanning without contrast material, then repeating the study with intravenous contrast enhancement. Whenever possible, the repeat scans should be taken at the same location as the unenhanced images. Comparing the slice with and without contrast enhancement facilitates accurate interpretation.

ORAL / RECTAL CONTRAST MEDIA PREPARATION

1.5-2% solution of iodine containing contrast media is used for bowel opacification. Ionic contrast media is routinely used since it is cheaper and risk of reaction with oral contrast media is very less. Preparations are available exclusively for oral route such as gastrograffin which are still cheaper. IV preparations also can be used for oral administration. The 60-76% contrast media available in the vial has to be diluted to obtain a solution of 1.5-2% solution.

Concentration available = 76%

Concentration required = 2%

Dilution required = 76/2 = 37.5 (approx. 40 times). It means that you may dilute any amount of 76% contast media to 40 times to give you approximately a 2% solution. Suppose we are to prepare 1000 ml of 2% solution. Add approximately 25 ml (1000/40 = 25 ml) of 76% contrast media in to 975 ml of water. Since the percentage of contrast media required need not be exactly 2% it can be formulated aproximately as follows. Take 1000 ml of water and add the calculated amount (1000/40 = 25 ml) of contrast media i.e. 25 ml in 1000 ml of water.

Total amount of diluted contrast media required	Amount of 76% contrast media to be added	Amount of 60% contrast media to be added
500	10	15
750	20	25
1000	25	33
1250	30	40
1500	35	50

1. Oral

Oral contrast media is essential for all studies involving gastrointestinal tract directly or indirectly. 1.5-2% diluted ionic contrast medium (gastrograffin) is usually used. Even though dilute barium can be used, it gives inconsistent results and commercial preparations are not easily available. 1500 ml may be given when full abdominal evaluation is required. 750-1000 ml is required for upper abdominal study. Always remember that contrast media is a bitter solution and mixing with beverages may help to make it at least partially palatable. After a loading dose of 300-400 ml oral, ingestion one glass may be given at an interval of 15 minutes to keep the entire bowel equally opacified. Tab metochlorpamide may be given (not routine) with first dose of oral contrast to hasten gastric emptying. For a full abdominal study oral contrast may be started 3 hours before the proposed time of study and for upper abdomen 1.5 hours before. Patients should be adequately informed about the role of oral contrast media, as many patients will be reluctant to drink large volume of oral contrast. Those with difficulty to swallow may be fed by the Ryle's tube.

2. Intravenous contrast (IV)

For examinations that require IV contrast enhancement, the history must include general allergy, asthma and history of reaction to drugs and contrast media as well as any renal complications. If the patient's chart is accessible, it is helpful to check laboratory reports for the most recent blood urea nitrogen and creatinine values. Those with high risk for reactions should be given prophylactic medication while giving appointment (described in the chapter on contrast media). So it is wise to elicit history for high risk at the time of appointment itself, which can avoid a postponement of the study.

The practice of obtaining written **consent** from the patient for the administration of intravenous contrast material is a common practice. Acquiring a signed consent form documents that the procedure and risks were discussed with the patient. The practice is not universally accepted. Opponents believe that the process of reading and signing a consent form often increases patient anxiety and increases the likelihood of an adverse reaction. Further, they believe that the forms offer little protection in cases of litigation. I do customarily obtain consent before contrast study. A test dose should be given 10 minutes before bolus injection and watched for signs or symptoms of adverse reaction.

3. Rectal

500 ml of 2% diluted contrast media should be given per rectal route via enema in all pelvic studies and when colonic pathologies area is of concern. This will enable us to visualize rectum, and invasion from other structures adequately. Air can be insufflated for negative contrast whenever positive contrast is contraindicated (e.g. CT angio).

4. Vaginal

Vagina may be filled with gauze immersed in dilute contrast media in all parous women undergoing pelvic evaluation. This helps to differentiate the relationship of different structures in relation to vagina.

5. Intrathecal

Intrathecal contrast is used when subarachnoid opacification is required for the study of spinal canal and CSF rhinorrhoea evaluation. Contrast is instilled via lumbar (common) or cervical routes. Non-ionic contrast media preferably iohexol is used. The quantity depends on when and what areas are scanned. For immediate scanning low dose myelography is enough (5 ml for lumbar and 7 ml for cervical CT).

PATIENT POSITIONING

For study of head & neck, chest, abdomen and spine, head is introduced first in to the gantry (Head first). For the study of extremities, feet are first introduced (Feet first). It important to enter head/feet first in the computed patient data, because if wrongly entered patient side will be wrongly displayed.

PATIENT INSTRUCTIONS

All patients undergoing CT scan should be explained briefly about the steps involved in the scanning briefly. The importance of keeping him at rest and obeying breathing instructions are stressed. It is better to demonstrate breath-holding and check with the patient how many seconds he can hold the breath without much discomfort. I do suggest th technologists to use a coaching procedure to increase the length of breath-hold especially for spiral study. This coaching requires the patient to take several deep breaths before taking one final breath and holding it for the maximum possible time, then exhaling slowly. For abdominal study holding the breath in mid-inspiration is quite enough but for chest deep inspiration is required. Patient should be instructed to keep the same amount of breath every time to avoid misregistration. In chest studies deep inspiration is essential.

SCANOGRAM

The preliminary image each scanner produces has many names. Siemens refers to this image as a topogram; General Electric calls it a scout; Toshiba calls it a scanogram. Scanogram is used for defining the limits of the scan and also marking each slice level and thickness. In all routine studies, a digital X-ray image, or scout, is acquired before scanning. The optimal scout includes all areas to be scanned and therefore ensures that the anatomy to be imaged is within the range of the system. A patient may lie out of the scanable range if he/she is positioned too close to the end of the scanning table. Regardless of the type of scanner used, it is imperative that the operator input the correct directional instructions before scanning. This procedure requires indicating whether the patient is placed head or feet first into the gantry and whether he is lying supine, prone, or in the decubitus position. If the operator accurately enters this information into the system, the software correctly annotates the image as to left-right and anterior-posterior orientation. It is a prerequisite for any scan series. Scout can be AP or lateral. Before obtaining scout make sure that the gantry tilt angle is zero. Also see whether scout scan range is 250/350/400 depending on FOV.

REFERENCE LINE / POINT

After the scout image is obtained, the operator selects the location of cross-sectional slices. Most scan procedures rely on beginning and ending landmarks that can be seen on the scout image. With some protocols, it is impossible to use readily identifiable landmarks. In these cases, the operator must make an educated guess, take one image to check the accuracy of the guess, and then proceed. This procedure is often helpful when scanning the adrenal gland. In this situation, a thin slice is required at the level of the adrenals. However, from the scout image, there is no way to predict with any degree of accuracy where the adrenals lie within the abdomen. Obviously, checking the first image before proceeding slows down the examination process, but the delay is unavoidable.

SCAN EXTENT

The scan extent of each study is decided by the area of interest in that particular case. Adequate provision should be given to study the upper and lower end of the region adequately.

SCAN PLANE

The technologist dealing with any imaging procedure should have thorough understanding of the common terminologies and imaging planes. Incorrect or impartial understanding of the terminology can cause lot of confusion.

The terms anterior and ventral refer to movement forward i.e. toward the face. Posterior and dorsal are equivalents used to describe movement toward the back surface of the body. Inferior refers to movement toward the feet and is synonymous with caudal. Superior defines movement toward the head and is used interchangably with the term cranial. Lateral refers to movement toward the sides of the body and medial refers to movement toward the midline of the body. The terms distal and proximal are most often used in referring to extremities. Distal refers to movement toward the ends. Proximal, which is the opposite of distal, may be defined as situated near the point of attachment.

To help visualize the imaginary body planes, it is helpful to think of large sheets of glass cutting through the body in various ways. All sheets of glass that are parallel to the floor are called horizontal, or transverse planes. Those

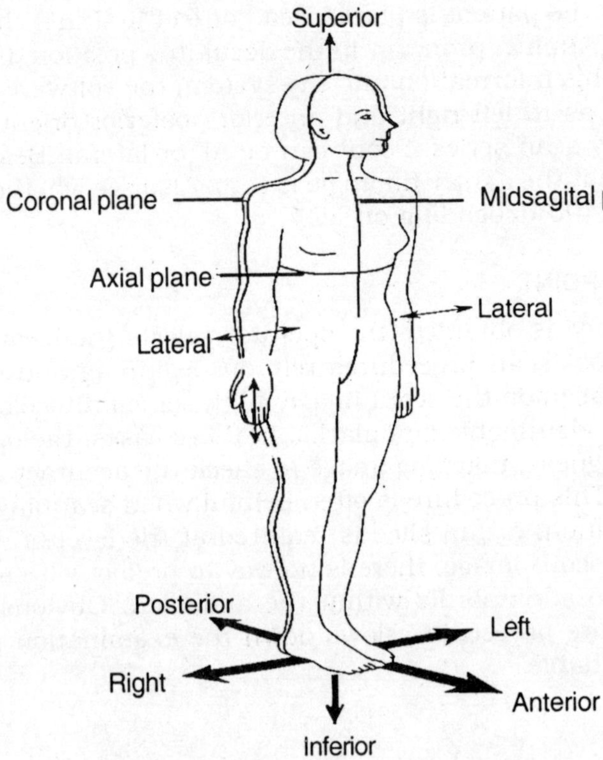

Fig. 11.1. Body planes

that stand perpendicular to the floor are called vertical or longitudinal planes. An imaginary plane that divides the body into anterior and posterior sections is the coronal plane. The sagittal plane divides the body into right and left sections. The sagittal plane that is located directly in the center, making left and right sections of equal size, is appropriately referred to as the median or mid-sagittal plane. A parasagittal plane is located to either the left or the right of the midline. Axial planes are cross-sectional planes that divide the body into upper and lower sections. Oblique planes are sheets of glass that are slanted and lie at an angle to one of the three standard planes.

Changing imaging planes in CT provides additional information. Changing the imaging plane from axial to coronal is indicated for two distinct reasons. The primary reason is when the anatomy lies vertically rather than horizontally. The ethmoid sinuses are an example of this principle. Because the ethmoid turbinates lay predominantly in the vertical plane, images taken in an axial plane show only sections of the anatomy, with no view of the entire ethmoid complex. The second indication for scanning in a different plane is to reduce artifacts created by surrounding structures. For this reason, the coronal plane is preferred for scanning the pituitary gland.

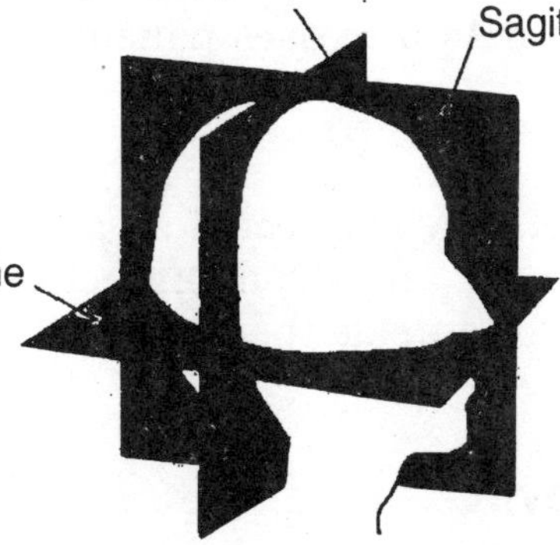

Fig. 11.2. Body planes

There are two methods of achieving a coronal position for head scanning. One is to place the patient prone on the scanning table and ask the patient to extend the chin forward. An alternative approach is to place the patient supine and ask him to drop his head back as far as possible. If the patient cannot extend the neck fully, the gantry may be angled to obtain a more coronal plane. The image obtained in either the prone or the supine coronal position is essentially the same. The preferred position involves several factors, including patient comfort, radiologist preference, and the effect of gravity on anatomic structures.

12. SCAN PARAMETERS

1. Algorithm

There are three standard settings for algorithm: smooth (soft), standard and sharp. In these the edges are highlighted or softened. Image sharpness is increased or decreased and image noise is increased or decreased in the reconstructed image. Selection of algorithm is done by using "Convolution Kernals " (CK). Usually scans are done in standard algorithm. Reconstruction in soft algorithm is useful when images are reconstructed for 3D imaging. Sharp algorithms are selected when sharpness of the image is of prime importance as in bone and lung.

2. kV

It determines the maximum possible energy of radiation. Higher kV is selected when thick /dense part is scanned and lower kv for small parts. Usual kV settings are 120 and 140.

3. mA

The higher the mAs the higher the number of photons reaching the detector. Image noise in inversely proportional the mAs used. Hence high mAs have to be used when thick part is scanned and when thin slices are used to reduce noise. However increase in mAs increases patient dose too.

4. Scan field of view (SFOV)

Large or small scan field of view is selected as per the part scanned. Usual SFOV ranges are 25 cm, 35 cm, and 45 cm respectively for brain, thorax, and abdomen. Part of the patient outside the scan field may cause inaccuracies called out of field artifact.

5. Display field of view (DFOV)

Display field of view is the region of the image selected for display in the monitor. Even if we have selected larger scan field of view always reconstruct the image in smaller display field of view to just encompass the region scanned. This will provide larger image with better resolution.

6. Slice thickness and table feed

When slice thickness is reduced the number of quanta within the slice is also reduced. When the slice thickness is reduced to half, the noise increases to 1.4 times. Scan protocols in which the slice thickness and spacing are equal are known as contiguous. Scans are not always taken in a contiguous fashion, however, in some cases, spacing is less than slice thickness. This practice results in overlapping images. Images may be overlapped if more slices are desired in a small area, such as the intervertebral disk space.

7. Scan time

It is always better to scan using the shortest time possible to avoid motion artifacts, to reduce total scan time, and to scan with good contrast enhancement. However, scan time may have to be increased to obtain adequate mAs to provide noiseless image in machines with lower mA settings.

13. IMAGE REVIEW

Image review by radiologists or at least by technologists is essential before the patient is shifted from the table. The purpose of image review is to check and decide whether

1. Area of interest is fully covered or not
2. Scan field of view was correct or not
3. Is there any pathology
4. Thin additional sections are required or not
5. Contrast study is essential or not.

14. POST PROCESSING

1. Recon algorithm

When the images are retrospectively reconstructed, appropriate algorithm has to be chosen. For example chest scan may be done in standard algorithm and the images can be retrospectively reconstructed in sharp algorithm using lung filter. Original images in standard algorithm can be used for mediastinal evaluation and reconstructed images for lung evaluation.

2. Recon FOV

Even if the scan was done using larger FOV, when images are reconstructed we may choose a smaller FOV just to encompass the body of concerned region. Targeted reconstruction with very small FOV to just include the pathological small area is very useful especially in lungs, temporal bones etc.

3. Filter

Appropriate filters like lung, bone, etc should be used whenever available. The terminologies for variable filters are different depending on the make.

4. Motion correction

Whenever there is suspicion of motion artifacts distorting the image and repeat scans are not possible, motion correction software may give a better image. It should be remembered that it is not as efficient as repeating the scan.

5. Multiplanar reconstruction (MPR)

Wherever possible provide multiplanar reformations in sagittal, parasagittal and coronal planes.

6. 3D Reformation

Scan protocols should be modified when 3D reformation is foreseen.

15. PHOTOGRAPHY

1. Cross-reference

After completion of a study, it is a standard procedure to include a scout image that is cross-referenced by lines. These lines represent the location of each cross-sectional image. Cross-reference is very helpful for location identification and planning of surgery.

2. Window settings

The CT value scale is up to 4000 HU. But the monitor has only 256 gray level scales. The human eye can differentiate only about 40 levels of brightness. The procedure of selecting the most diagnostically relevant region of HU scales for a given examination and distributing the CT scale among the 256 gray levels is called windowing. Window centering is specifying as to which CT value is to be displayed at the middle of the gray scale. The window width determines the region of interest. All CT values below this range are displayed black and those above this as white.

3. Printing format

It is always better to use less number of images in a film. However, we have to think about economy also and hence optimization of the number of images to be printed in a film is essential. This may vary from center to center.

16. SPECIAL NOTE

There are so many instructions and special precautions to be remembered in different scans. They cannot be discussed in one heading. The technologists should have thorough knowledge of these aspects.

CHAPTER 12

Conventional CT Scan Protocols

PROTOCOLS FOR CT HEAD AND NECK

CCT-BRAIN PLAIN

INDICATIONS	: Headache, cerebrovascular, accidents, hydrocephalus, adult onset, seizures, trauma
ENHANCEMENT TECHNIQUES	
• Oral	: Nil
• IV-ml/Delay	: Nil
PATIENT POSITIONING	: Head First/Supine
SCANOGRAM	: Skull lateral up to C3
REFERENCE LINE	: Parallel to OM line
SCAN REGION	: Base of skull to vertex
SCAN PLANE	: Axial
SCAN PARAMETERS	
• Algorithm/kV/mA	: STD/140 kV/120 mA
• SFOV/Time	: 25 cm/3 sec for infratentorial and 2 sec for supratentorial
• Slice thickness	: 5/5 for infratentorial and 10/10 for supratentorial
IMAGE REVIEW	: Look for small lesions and obtain thin section in the concerned region
POST PROCESSING	
• Recon mode/FOV	: STD/19 cm

- Filter/Motion correction : STD/if needed
- Reformation/3D : Nil/Nil

PHOTOGRAPHY

- Window settings : 120/40 for post fossa
  : 100/35 for supratentorial
- Printing format : 17 × 14 -12 on 1

SPECIAL NOTE : mAs can be reduced when small children and infants are studied

CCT-HEAD FOR TRAUMA

INDICATIONS : Acute or chronic trauma.

ENHANCEMENT TECHNIQUES

- Oral : Nil
- IV-ml/ Delay : Nil

PATIENT POSITIONING : Head First/Supine

SCANOGRAM : Skull lateral up to C7

REFERENCE LINE : Parallel to OM line

SCAN REGION : Base of skull to vertex

SCAN PLANE : Axial

SCAN PARAMETERS

- Algorithm/kV/mA : STD/140kV/120mA
- SFOV/Time : 25/3 sec for infratentorial and 2 sec for supratentorial
- Slice thickness : 5/5 for infratentorial and 10/10 for supratentorial

IMAGE REVIEW : Look for small lesions and obtain thin section in the concerned region.

SPECIAL INSTRUCTION : Always include zygomatic arch as it is a common site for fracture

POST PROCESSING

- Recon algorithm/FOV : Bone /20 cm
- Filter/Motion correction : Sharp/if needed
- MPR/3D : Nil/Nil

PHOTOGRAPHY

- Window settings : 120/40 for post fossa
  : 100/35 for supratentorial
- Printing format : 17 × 14 - 12 on 1 for brain

	: 17 × 14 -12 on 1 for bone Provide scout film with cross reference

CCT-BRAIN CONTRAST

INDICATION	: Headache, tumour, seizures, meningitis, vascular malformation, abscess, granuloma
ENHANCEMENT TECHNIQUES	
• Oral	: Nil
• IV-ml/ Delay	: 30-50 ml hand injection/immediately after injection
PATIENT POSITIONING	: Head First/Supine
SCANOGRAM	: Skull lateral up to C3
REFERENCE LINE	: Parallel to OM line
SCAN REGION	: Base of skull to vertex
SCAN PLANE	: Axial
SCAN PARAMETERS	
• Algorithm/kV/mA	: STD/140 kV/120 mA
• SFOV/Time	: 25/3 sec for infratentorial and 2 sec for supratentorial
• Slice thickness	: 5/5 for infratentorial and 10/10 for supratentorial
IMAGE REVIEW	: Look for small lesions and obtain thin section in the concerned region.
POST PROCESSING	
• Recon algorithm/FOV	: STD/19 cm
• Filter/Motion correction	: STD/if needed
• MPR/3D	: Nil/Nil
PHOTOGRAPHY	
• Window settings	: 120/40 for post fossa
	: 100/35 for supratentorial
• Printing format	: 17 × 14 -12 on 1
SPECIAL NOTE	: In patient suspected to have CP angle lesion 2 mm additional axial sections may be obtained through IAC and reconstruction and photography of the same region in bone window is recommended to show IAC expansion/erosion. In children contrast dose can be calculated as 2 ml/kg

CCT-BRAIN AND SELLA POST CONTRAST

INDICATIONS : Parasellar lesions, pituitary lesions, cavernous sinus lesions

ENHANCEMENT TECHNIQUES

- Oral : Nil
- IV-ml/Delay : 30-50 ml hand injection/scan immediately after injection

PATIENT POSITIONING : Head First/Supine for brain prone for coronal scan of sella

SCANOGRAM : Skull lateral up to C3

REFERENCE LINE : Parallel to OM line

SCAN REGION : Base of skull to vertex axial 1 cm anterior to ant clinoid 1 cm post to dorsum sella

SCAN PLANE : Axial brain and sella coronalsella

SCAN PARAMETERS

- Algorithm/kV/mA : STD/140 kV/120 mA
- SFOV/Time : 25 cm/3 sec for infratentorial and sella, 2 sec for supratentorial
- Slice thickness : 5/5 for infratentorial 3/3 for sella and 10/10 for supratentorial 3 mm contiguous coronal scan for sella

IMAGE REVIEW : Look for small hypodense lesions in pituitary.

POST PROCESSING

- Recon algorithm/FOV : Nil/19 cm for brain and 10 mm for sella
- Filter/Motion correction : STD/if needed
- Reformation/3D : Sagittal for sella/Nil

PHOTOGRAPHY

- Window settings : 120/40 for post. fossa
  : 100/35 for supratentorial
- Printing format : 17 × 14 -12 on 1 for brain

CCT- SELLA CONTRAST

INDICATIONS : Parasellar lesions, pituitary lesions, cavernous sinus lesions

ENHANCEMENT TECHNIQUES

- Oral : Nil

• IV-ml/Delay	: 30 ml for axial and 30 ml for coronal/Hand injection/Scan is done immediately after injection
PATIENT POSITIONING	: Head First/Supine for axial and prone for coronal scan
SCANOGRAM	: Skull lateral
REFERENCE LINE	: Axial parallel to floor of sella and coronal perpendicular to it
SCAN REGION	: From 1 cm anterior to anterior clinoid/ lesion to 1 cm posterior to dorsum sella/ lesion
SCAN PLANE	: Axial and coronal
SCAN PARAMETERS	
• Algorithm/ kV/mA	: STD/140 kV/120 mA
• SFOV/Time	: 25 cm/3 sec
• Slice thickness	: 3/3 for axial and coronal
IMAGE REVIEW	: Look for small hypodense lesions in pituitary. See whether the entire lesion is covered by the scan
POST PROCESSING	
• Recon algorithm/FOV	: STD and bone/19 cm for brain and 10 mm for sella
• Filter/motion correction	: STD and bone/if needed
• Reformation/3D	: Multiple sagittal and parasagittal for sella including cavernous sinuses/Nil
PHOTOGRAPHY	
• Window settings	: 300/40 for pituitary
	: 3500/700 for bone
• Printing format	: 17 × 14 - 9 on 1 for axial
	: 17 × 14 - 12 on 1 for coronal including bone window

CCT–ORBIT

INDICATIONS	: Proptosis, loss of vision, trauma, inflammation, infection, mass
ENHANCEMENT TECHNIQUES	
• Oral	: Nil
• IV-ml/ Delay	: 30 ml for axial and 30 ml for coronal. Hand injection. Scan is done immediately after injection

PATIENT POSITIONING	: Head first/supine for axial and prone for coronal scan
SCANOGRAM	: Skull lateral
REFERENCE LINE	: Axial parallel to the Reid's baseline and coronal perpendicular to it
SCAN REGION	: Supra- to infraorbital margin for axial and ant. orbital margin to tuberculum sella.
SCAN PLANE	: Axial and coronal
SCAN PARAMETERS	
• Algorithm/kV/mA	: STD/140 kV/120 mA
• SFOV/Time	: 25/3 sec
• Slice thickness	: 3/3 for axial and coronal
SPECIAL INSTRUCTIONS	: Contrast not required for trauma
	: If direct coronal not possible obtain thinner contiguous axial sections for coronal reformation
IMAGE REVIEW	: See whether optic canal is well visualized or not
POST PROCESSING	
• Recon algorithm/FOV	: STD and bone/20 cm
• Filter/Motion correction	: STD and bone/if needed
• Reformation/3D	: Multiple coronal if only axial images are obtained/May be done in trauma cases
PHOTOGRAPHY	
• Window settings	: 200/40 for pituitary
	: 3500/700 for bone
• Printing format	: 17 × 14 -16 on 1 for axial including bone window
	: 17 × 14-16 on 1 for coronal including bone window
SPECIAL NOTE	: Ried's baseline is 10° from the OM line, as it usually parallels the optic nerve. CECT does not greatly increase the visualization of the intraorbital vessels or other structures, as there is already inherent contrast between the orbital structure and retro- orbital fat. CECT is usually reserved for identifying the vascular lesions such as aneurysms/AVMs/meningiomas of the para-

sellar region. Coronal images are useful in assessing the size of optic nerves and in evaluating the floor and roof of the orbit especially in case of trauma.

CCT- TEMPORAL BONE

INDICATIONS : Hearing loss, 7th nerve palsy, congenital anomalies, trauma, tumour, cholesteotoma, otitis media, otosclerosis

ENHANCEMENT TECHNIQUES

- Oral : Nil
- IV-ml/Delay : NIl

PATIENT POSITIONING : Head first/Supine for axial and prone for coronal scan

SCANOGRAM : Skull lateral

REFERENCE LINE : Axial scan done with 30 degree upward angulation to Ried's baseline. (This line is parallel to the lateral semi-circular canal and displays the temporal bone structures to the best advantage. Coronal scan is obtained at 120 degree above the anthropological baseline)

SCAN REGION : For 3 cm with EOM as center.

SCAN PLANE : Axial and coronal

SCAN PARAMETERS

- Algorithm/ kV/mA : Bone/140 kV/140 mA
- SFOV/Time : 25/3sec
- Slice thickness : 1/2 for axial and coronal

SPECIAL INSTRUCTIONS : Contrast may be required in case of glomus jugulare and other vascular and non-vascular tumours.

IMAGE REVIEW : See whether optic canal is well visualized or not

POST PROCESSING

- Recon algorithm/FOV : Bone (targetted recon for both temporal bone seperatly is optional)/20 cm
- Filter/ Motion correction : Sharp/if needed
- Reformation/3D : Multiple coronal if only axial images are obtained/May be done in trauma cases

PHOTOGRAPHY

- Window settings : 4000/700
- Printing format : 17 × 14 - 16 on 1 for axial
  : 17 × 14 - 16 on 1 for coronal

CCT-TEMPERO MANDIBULAR JOINTS

INDICATIONS : Trauma, infection, tumour, trismus, TM joint abnormalities

ENHANCEMENT TECHNIQUES

- Oral : Nil
- IV-ml/Delay : Nil

PATIENT POSITIONING : Head first/Supine for axial and prone for coronal

SCANOGRAM : Skull lateral

REFERENCE LINE : Axial parallel to hard palate coronal parallel to the ramus of the mandible

SCAN REGION : From 1 cm above and 1 cm below the joints for axial and full coverage of the joint in coronal.

SCAN PLANE : Axial and coronal

SCAN PARAMETERS

- Algorithm /kV/mA : Bone/140 kV/140 mA
- SFOV/DFOV : 25/20
- Slice thickness/time : 3/5 for axial and coronal/3 sec

SPECIAL INSTRUCTIONS : Open mouth.

IMAGE REVIEW : Nil

POST PROCESSING

- Recon algorithm/FOV : Bone (targeted recon for both TM joint is optional)/20 cm
- Filter/Motion correction : Sharp/if needed
- Reformation/3D : Sagittal through each condyle/may be done.

PHOTOGRAPHY

- Window settings : 3500/700 for bone
- Printing format : 17 × 14 -12 on 1 for axial.
  : 17 × 14-12 on 1 for coronal

CCT-CORONAL SCREENING SINUS CT

INDICATIONS	: Screening before FESS. Chronic sinusitis not responding to conventional treatment.
ENHANCEMENT TECHNIQUES	
• Oral	: Nil
• IV-ml/Delay	: Nil
PATIENT POSITIONING	: Head First/Prone
SCANOGRAM	: Skull lateral
REFERANCE LINE	: Perpendicular to the hard palate
SCAN REGION	: Ant frontal sinus to post sphenoid sinus.
SCAN PLANE	: Coronal
SCAN PARAMETERS	
• Algorithm/kV/mA	: Sharp/140 kV/140 mA
• SFOV/Time	: 25 cm/2 sec
• Slice thickness	: 3/3 for OM complex and 5/5 for posterior part
SPECIAL INSTRUCTIONS	: Pretreatment with antibiotics and antihistamines preferred. Ask the patient to sneeze out completely the secretions before the scan.
IMAGE REVIEW	: See for visualization of infundibulum, optic canal etc
POST PROCESSING	
• Recon algorithm/FOV	: Detail/15 cm
• Filter/Motion correction	: Sharp/Nil
• Reformation/3D	: Sagittal/Nil
PHOTOGRAPHY	
• Window settings	: 2000/200 may be taken for preliminary setting and adjust the window so that the infundibulum clearly, the same setting can be used for 3500/700 for optic canal and sella.
• Printing format	: 17 × 14 -16 on 1

CCT-CORONAL SINUS CT FOR TRAUMA

INDICATIONS	: Sinusitis, trauma, tumour, polyps.
ENHANCEMENT TECHNIQUES	
• Oral	: Nil
• IV-ml/ Delay	: Nil

PATIENT POSITIONING : Head First/Prone
SCANOGRAM : Skull lateral
REFERENCE LINE : Perpendicular to hard palate
SCAN REGION : From anterior to nasal bone to post sphenoid sinus.
SCAN PLANE : Coronal
SCAN PARAMETERS
- Algorithm/kV/mA : STD/140 kV/140 mA
- SFOV/Time : 25/2 sec
- Slice thickness/Time : 5/5 mm

SPECIAL INSTRUCTIONS : Contrast may be useful in tumour cases
IMAGE REVIEW : Nil
POST PROCESSING
- Recon algorithm/FOV : Bone/15 cm
- Filter/Motion correction : Sharp/Nil
- Reformation/3D : Sagittal/may be done

PHOTOGRAPHY
- Window settings : 280/40 for soft tissue.
  : 3500/700 for bone window.
- Printing format : 17 × 14 -16 on 1

SPECIAL NOTE : This is the recommended plane of scan for orbital blowout fractures

CCT- BRAIN AND PNS SCREENING

INDICATIONS : Headache trauma, sinusitis, tumour,
ENHANCEMENT TECHNIQUES
- Oral : Nil
- IV-ml/ Delay : May be required in tumour cases

PATIENT POSITIONING : Head First/Supine.
SCANOGRAM : Skull lateral
REFERENCE LINE : OM line
SCAN REGION : Base of skull to vertex for brain
: For sinuses from hard palate to top of frontal sinuses
SCAN PLANE : Supine
SCAN PARAMETERS
- Algorithm/kV/mA : STD/140 kV/140 mA
- SFOV/Time : 25/2sec

• Slice thickness.	: 5/5 for posterior fossa, 10/10 for supratentorial brain, 5/5 for sinuses.
SPECIAL INSTRUCTIONS	: Contrast may be usefull in tumour cases
IMAGE REVIEW	: Nil
POST PROCESSING	
• Recon algorithm/FOV	: Bone for trauma cases/15 cm
• Filter/Motion correction	: Sharp for trauma/May be required
• Reformation/3D	: NIL/may be done
PHOTOGRAPHY	
• Window settings	: Usual settings for brain. 280/40 soft tissue PNS. 2000/200 for Bone window
• Printing format	: 17 × 14 -16 on 1 for brain. 17 × 14 -16 on 1 for PNS
SPECIAL NOTE	: This test is usually asked by the ENT surgeons when the cause of headache is unknown and no localizing signs are present. It is done as a general screening procedure to reveal any obvious pathology in the PNS or Brain

CCT- NECK SURVEY

INDICATIONS	: Lymph node screening.
ENHANCEMENT TECHNIQUES	
• Oral	: Nil
• IV-ml/Delay	: 50 ml immediately after injection.
PATIENT POSITIONING	: Head First/Supine.
PATIENT INSTRUCTIONS	:
SCANOGRAM	: Neck lateral.
REFERANCE LINE	: Parallel to vertebral end plate
SCAN REGION	: Base of skull to thoracic inlet.
SCAN PLANE	: Axial
SCAN PARAMETERS	
• Algorithm/ kV/mA	: STD/120 kV/140 mA
• SFOV/Time	: 25 cm/2 sec
• Slice thickness	: 5/7 mm
SPECIAL INSTRUCTIONS	: Gantry angulation appropriate to exclude dental artifacts.
IMAGE REVIEW	: Nil

POST PROCESSING
- Recon algorithm/FOV : Nil/Nil
- Filter/Motion correction : Nil/Nil
- MPR/3D : Nil/Nil

PHOTOGRAPHY
- Window settings : 240/40 soft tissue PNS.
- Printing format : 17 × 14 -16 on 1

CCT–PHARYNX

INDICATIONS : Neoplasm, inflammation.

ENHANCEMENT TECHNIQUES
- Oral : Nil
- IV-ml/Delay : 50 ml immediately after injection.

PATIENT POSITIONING : Head first/Supine.

PATIENT INSTRUCTIONS : Patient is instructed not to swallow during scanning

SCANOGRAM : Neck lateral.

REFERENCE LINE : Parallel to vertebral end plate

SCAN REGION : Base of skull to hyoid bone.

SCAN PLANE : Axial. Coronal study is useful in nasopharynx

SCAN PARAMETERS
- Algorithm/ kV/mA : STD/120 kV/140 mA
- SFOV/Time : 25/2 sec
- Slice thickness : 5/7 mm

SPECIAL INSTRUCTIONS : Appropriate gantry angulation to exclude dental artifacts.

IMAGE REVIEW : Nil

POST PROCESSING
- Recon algorithm/FOV : STD/Include neck in case of cervical adenopathy
- Filter/Motion correction : STD/If needed
- MPR/3D : Sagittal and coronal/NIL

PHOTOGRAPHY
- Window settings : 240/40
- Printing format : 17 × 14 -16 on 1

CCT–LARYNX

INDICATIONS : Neoplasm, inflammation.
Cong lesions.

ENHANCEMENT TECHNIQUES
- Oral : Nil
- IV-ml/ Delay : 50 ml immediately after injection.

PATIENT POSITIONING : Head First, supine

PATIENT INSTRUCTIONS : Patient is instructed not to swallow during scanning

SCANOGRAM : Neck lateral.

REFERENCE LINE : Parallel to vertebral endplate

SCAN REGION : Epiglotis to below cricoid cartilage.

SCAN PLANE : Axial

SCAN PARAMETERS
- Algorithm/ kV/mA : STD/120 kV/140 mA
- SFOV/Time : 25/2 sec
- Slice thickness : 3/5 mm. Additional 1 mm sections may be obtained for vocal cord

SPECIAL INSTRUCTIONS : Valsalva maneuver and phonation are useful for airway evaluation. Patient is instructed not to swallow and breath.

IMAGE REVIEW : Nil

POST PROCESSING
- Recon algorithm/FOV : STD/15 cm.
- Filter/Motion correction : STD/If needed.
- MPR/3D : Sagittal and coronal/Nil

PHOTOGRAPHY
- Window settings : 240/40
- Printing format : 17 × 14 -16 on 1

CCT- IN CSF LEAK

INDICATIONS : Fracture base skull, CSF leak

ENHANCEMENT TECHNIQUES
- Oral : Nil
- IV-ml/Delay :
- Intrathecal : 7-10 ml

PATIENT POSITIONING : Head first, Prone
SCANOGRAM : Skull lateral.
REFERANCE LINE : Perpendicular to hard palate
SCAN REGION : Root of the nose to clivus.
SCAN PLANE : Coronal. Axial scan may be obtained when there is suspicion of CSF leakage at the temporal bones.

SCAN PARAMETERS
- Algorithm/kV/mA : Bone/120 kV/140 mA
- SFOV/Time : 25/2 sec
- Slice thickness : 3/3 mm. Additional 1 mm sections may be obtained at the region of suspicion.

SPECIAL INSTRUCTIONS : CT Cisternography may be necessary if plain HRCT and MR cisternography is inconclusive.

IMAGE REVIEW : Look for bone defect, CSF column extending across bone defect extracranially, herniation of brain or meninges across the bone defect or with air communicating from the PNS intracranially. On CT cisternography a contrast column extending from intracranial compartment would be diagnostic for CSF fistula.

POST PROCESSING
- Recon algorithmFOV : Bone/15 cm
- Filter/Motion correction : Sharp/If needed.
- MPR/3D : Sagittal /NIL

PHOTOGRAPHY
- Window settings : 2000/300
- Printing format : 17 × 14 -16 on 1

PROTOCOLS FOR CT CHEST

CCT–CHEST PLAIN SCREENING

INDICATIONS : Screening for subtle neoplasm or inflammation

ENHANCEMENT TECHNIQUES
- Oral : Nil
- IV-ml/Delay : NIL

PATIENT POSITIONING	: Head First, supine
PATIENT INSTRUCTIONS	: Patient is instructed to hold the breath in full inspiration and to keep the level of inspiration same at all sections
SCANOGRAM	: Chest AP
SCAN REGION	: Apex to lung base
REFERENCE LINE	: Sternal notch
SCAN PLANE	: Axial
SCAN PARAMETERS	
• Algorithm/ kV/mA	: STD/120 kV/160 mA
• SFOV/Time	: 35/1-2 sec
• Slice thickness	: 10/10
SPECIAL INSTRUCTIONS	: If mediastinal or lung masses are visualized contrast study may be required
IMAGE REVIEW	:
POST PROCESSING	
• Recon algorithm/FOV	: Bone/30 cm depending on patient size.
• Filter/Motion correction	: Lungs/If needed.
• MPR/3D	: Nil/Nil
PHOTOGRAPHY	
• Window settings	: 1500/700 For lungs : 350/50 For mediastinum.
• Printing format	: 17 × 14 -16 on 1 for lungs
	: 17 × 14 -16 on 1 for mediastinum

CCT–CHEST FOR MASS LESIONS

INDICATIONS	: Lung, mediastinal, pleural or esophageal mass lesions, inflammatory, and congenital lesions. empyema, chest wall pathologies
ENHANCEMENT TECHNIQUES	
• Oral	: Nil
• IV-ml/Delay	: 50 ml immediately after injection.
PATIENT POSITIONING	: Head First, Supine
PATIENT INSTRUCTIONS	: Patient is instructed to hold the breath in full inspiration and keep the level of inspiration same at all levels

SCANOGRAM : Chest AP.
REFERENCE LINE : Sternal notch.
SCAN REGION : Lung apex to adrenal levels.
SCAN PLANE : Axial
SCAN PARAMETERS
- Algorithm/kV/mA : STD/120 kV/160 mA
- SFOV/Time : 35/1-2 sec
- Slice thickness : 10/10 plain. 10/10 from apex to 25 mm above carina. 5/5 from 25 mm above carina to 60 mm below carina. 10/10 from 60 mm below carina to adrenal level

SPECIAL INSTRUCTIONS : Breath holding in deep inspiration and maintain the same level of inspiration at all slices should be advised and demonstrated. Oral contrast may be given in cases of esophageal pathology. Extend the study to the level of celiac axis in cases of esophageal malignancy. Additional prone scanning may be done in cases of fungal ball in a cavity.

IMAGE REVIEW :
POST PROCESSING
- Recon algorithm FOV : Sharp/30 cm depending on patient size.
- Filter/Motion correction : Lung/If needed.
- MPR/3D : Nil/Nil

PHOTOGRAPHY
- Window settings : 1500/-700 for lungs. 350/50 for mediastinum.
- Printing format : 17 × 14 -12 on 1 for lungs 2 films
  : 17 × 14 -16 on 1 for mediastinum

CCT–HRCT LUNGS

INDICATIONS : Hemoptysis, ILD, miliary TB, COPD, emphysema, bronchiectasis, lymphangitis carcinomatosis etc

ENHANCEMENT TECHNIQUES
- Oral : Nil
- IV-ml/Delay : Nil

PATIENT POSITIONING	: Head first, Supine
PATIENT INSTRUCTIONS	: Patient is instructed to hold the breath in full inspiration and keep the level of inspiration same at all levels
SCANOGRAM	: Chest AP
REFEReNCE LINE	: Sternal notch
SCAN REGION	: Lung apex to base
SCAN PLANE	: Axial
SCAN PARAMETERS	
• Algorithm/kV/mA	: STD/120 kV/200 mA (high mAs)
• SFOV/Time	: 35/1-2 sec (shortest possible)
• Slice thickness	: 1-2 mm/10 mm (thinnest possible)
	: 5/5 for hila advised when evaluating for hemoptysis.
SPECIAL INSTRUCTIONS	: Breath holding in deep inspiration and maintain the same level of inspiration in all slices should be advised and demonstrated. Additional prone scanning may be required to demonstrate dependent density.
IMAGE REVIEW	: Expiratory scans are useful to differentiate mosaic perfusion from air trapping. It may be done at three levels—aortic arch, carina, and two centimeters above the right dome of diaphragm.
POST PROCESSING	
• Recon algorithm/FOV	: Sharp/30 cm depending on patient size.
• Filter/Motion correction	: Lung/Yes
• MPR/3D	: Nil/Nil
PHOTOGRAPHY	
• Window settings	: 600-700/1500 may be used routinely for lungs. 500-700/2000 pleuroparenchymal abnormalities. 800-900/500 for documenting emphysema. 350/50 for mediastinum.
• Printing format	: 17 × 14 – 6-9 on 1 for lungs 2 films
	: 17 × 14 -16 on 1 for mediastinum
SPECIAL NOTE	: Low dose HRCT may be done to follow up cases using low mAs

PROTOCOLS FOR CT ABDOMEN

CECT (Contrast Enhanced Computed Tomography) is performed for angiographic information about vascular structures, gross cardiac anatomy, distinguishing tumours from blood vessels (during biopsy), to estimate blood flow to a lesion of solid or cystic type.

Liver : Each study has to be planned individually after review of clinical problem and the capabilities of the scanner. The opacification of GIT with oral contrast is standard for all studies of CT abdomen.

Spleen : Spleen being a highly vascular organ, it has peak levels of contrast enhancement shortly after aorta. On CECT, spleen displays CT value of 100-150 HU during arterial phase and 60-100 HU in venous phase.

Indications of CT kidney include:

1. To evaluate the renal masses when other imaging modalities have failed to yield the needed information.
2. To evaluate the juxtarenal lesion seen on IVU.
3. To evaluate a non functioning kidney at IVU to assess the size, shape and parenchyma thickness to detect the cause of obstruction and to pinpoint the size, height and extent of the disease process causing obstruction.
4. To document any congenital absence or variation.
5. To assess the extent of renal trauma.
6. To determine the cause of renal or perirenal calcification.
7. For guidance in PCN biopsy or aspiration.

CCT–WHOLE ABDOMINAL AND PELVIS SCREENING

INDICATIONS : Screening for neoplasm, infective foci,

ENHANCEMENT TECHNIQUES

- Oral : 1500 ml of 1.5-2% diluted contrast media may be given orally at a rate of 200 ml/15 minutes before the scan
- Rectal : 500 ml of 2% diluted contrast media may be given in all cases suspected to have pelvic or large bowel pathology.
- IV-ml/Delay : May be used if there is any relevant positive findings on plain CT

PATIENT POSITIONING : Head first, Supine

PATIENT INSTRUCTIONS : Patient is instructed to hold the breath

SCANOGRAM : Abdomen AP

REFERENCE LINE : Xiphisternum

SCAN REGION	: Dome of diaphragm to pubic symphysis
SCAN PLANE	: Axial
SCAN PARAMETERS	
• Algorithm/kV/mA	: STD/120 kV/140 mA
• SFOV/DFOV	: 45/35
• Slice thickness/Time	: 10 mm/10 mm/2 sec
SPECIAL INSTRUCTIONS	: Cluster scan facility if available may be used with 3-4 scan per breath followed by 15 sec breath time. Advised to maintain the same level of inspiration in all slices to avoid slice misregistration.
IMAGE REVIEW	: Look for any pathology and perform post IV contrast CT with thin sections (5 mm).
POST PROCESSING	
• Recon algorithm/FOV	: STD/35 depending on patient size.
• Filter/Motion correction	: STD/Yes
• MPR/3D	: Nil/Nil
PHOTOGRAPHY	
• Window settings	: 350/50
• Printing format	: 17 × 14 – 16 on 1-2 films

CCT- WHOLE ABDOMEN AND PELVIS P+C.

INDICATIONS	: Suspected primary, metastatic ca, neoplasia of GIT/urogenital system, PUO, trauma
ENHANCEMENT TECHNIQUES	
• Oral	: 1500 ml of 1.5-2% diluted contrast media may be given orally at a rate of 200 ml/15 minutes before the scan
• Rectal	: 500 ml of 2% diluted contrast media may be given in all cases suspected to have pelvic or large bowel pathology.
• IV-ml/ Delay	: 70 ml/scan immediately after hand injection.
PATIENT POSITIONING	: Head first, Supine
PATIENT INSTRUCTIONS	: Patient is instructed to hold the breath.
SCANOGRAM	: Abdomen AP.
REFERENCE LINE	: Xiphisternum
SCAN REGION	: Dome of diaphragm to pubic symphysis.

SCAN PLANE : Axial

SCAN PARAMETERS

- Algorithm/Kv/mA : STD/120 kV/140 mA
- SFOV/DFOV : 45/35
- Slice thickness : 10 mm/10 mm plain CT 5/7 mm from dome of diaphragm to lower pole of kidneys. 10/10 from lower pole of kidneys to iliac crest. 5/7 from iliac crest to pubic symphysis.
- Time : 2 sec

SPECIAL INSTRUCTIONS : Cluster scan facility if available may be used with 3-4 scan per breath followed by 15 sec breath time. Advised to maintain the same level of inspiration in all slices to avoid slice misregistration.

IMAGE REVIEW : Look for any pathology and perform post IV contrast CT with thin sections (5 mm).

POST PROCESSING

- Recon algorithm/FOV : STD/35 depending on patient size.
- Filter/Motion correction : STD/Yes
- MPR/3D : Nil/Nil

PHOTOGRAPHY

- Window settings : 350/50
- Printing format : 17 × 14 –16 on 1-2 films

CCT–UPPER ABDOMEN FOR HEPATOBILIATY SYSTEM P+C

INDICATIONS : Tumours and inflammation of liver pancreas,.stomach

ENHANCEMENT TECHNIQUES

- Oral : 1000 ml of 1.5-2% diluted contrast media may be given orally at a rate of 200 ml/15 minutes before the scan
- Rectal : Nil
- IV-ml/ Delay : 70 ml/scan immediately after hand injection.

PATIENT POSITIONING : Head first, Supine

PATIENT INSTRUCTIONS : Patient is instructed to hold the breath.

SCANOGRAM : Abdomen AP

REFERENCE POINT : Xiphisternum

SCAN REGION : Dome of diaphragm to iliac crest

SCAN PLANE : Axial

SCAN PARAMETERS

- Algorithm/ kV/mA : STD/120 kV/140 mA
- SFOV/Time : 45/2 sec
- Slice thickness : 10 mm/10 mm plain CT. 5/7 from dome of diaphragm to lower pole of kidneys: 10/10 from lower pole of kidneys to iliac crest.

SPECIAL INSTRUCTIONS : Cluster scan facility if available may be used with 3-4 scan per breath followed by 15 sec breath time. Advised to maintain the same level of inspiration in all slices to avoid slice misregistration.

IMAGE REVIEW : Look for any pathology. Additional special scanning for liver, pancreas or kidneys may be required. In that case follow the instructions given in the corresponding sections.

POST PROCESSING

- Recon algorithm/FOV : STD/35 depending on patient size.
- Filter/ Motion correction : STD/Yes
- MPR/3D : Nil/Nil

PHOTOGRAPHY

- Window settings : 350/50
- Printing format : 17 × 14 – 20 on 1 film for plain series
  : 17 × 14 – 20 on 2 film for contrast series.

CCT–DEDICATED STUDY FOR HEPATIC HEMANGIOMA

INDICATIONS : Strong suspicion of hepatic hemangioma for confirmation.

ENHANCEMENT TECHNIQUES

- Oral : 1000 ml of 1.5-2% diluted contrast media may be given orally at a rate of 200 ml/15 minutes before the scan
- Rectal : Nil
- IV-ml/Delay : 70 ml/scan immediately after hand injection.

PATIENT POSITIONING : Head first, Supine

PATIENT INSTRUCTIONS : Patient is instructed to hold the breath.

SCANOGRAM : Abdomen AP.

REFERENCE LINE	: Xiphisternum
SCAN REGION	: Dome of diaphragm to lower pole of liver.
SCAN PLANE	: Axial
SCAN PARAMETERS	
• Algorithm/kV/mA	: STD/120 kV/140 mA
• SFOV/Time	: 45/2 sec
• Slice thickness	: 10 mm/10 mm plain CT. Additional post contrast single location non-incremental scans are done through the centre of the lesion at 30 sec, 45, 1 m, 2 m, 3 m, 5 m, 10 m, 20 m
SPECIAL INSTRUCTIONS	: This dedicated study is done only to confirm hemangioma when the clinical and sonological suspicion is very high. But when the clinical situation demands differentiation of hemangioma from other hepatic tumous it is better to perform 5/7 post contrast study followed by additional delayed scan through the centre of the lesion.
IMAGE REVIEW	: Look for centripetal type of nodular contrast filling from the periphery gradually filling the entire lesion over a period which is diagnostic of hemangioma.
POST PROCESSING	
• Recon algorithm/FOV	: STD/35 depending on patient size.
• Filter/ Motion correction	: STD/Yes
• MPR/3D	: Nil/Nil
PHOTOGRAPHY	
• Window settings	: 350/50
• Printing format	: 17 × 14–20 on 1 film for plain series
	: 17 × 14–20 on 2 film for contrast series

CCT–UPPER ABDOMEN FOR PANCREAS

INDICATIONS	: Acute and chronic pancreatitis, pancreatic tumours, periampullary ca, cholangio ca
ENHANCEMENT TECHNIQUES	
• Oral	: 1000 ml of 1.5-2% diluted contrast media may be given orally at a rate of 200 ml/15 minutes before the scan

• Rectal	: Nil
• IV-ml/ Delay	: 100 ml/scan immediately after injection
PATIENT POSITIONING	: Head first, supine
PATIENT INSTRUCTIONS	: Patient is instructed to hold the breath.
SCANOGRAM	: Abdomen AP.
REFERENCE LINE	: Xiphisternum
SCAN REGION	: Dome of diaphragm to lower pole of kidney
SCAN PLANE	: Axial
SCAN PARAMETERS	
• Algorithm/kV/mA	: STD/120 kV/140 mA
• SFOV/Time	: 45/2 sec
• Slice thickness	: 10/10 precontrast. 5/7 from dome of diaphragm to just above pancreatic body. 3/5 from just above pancreatic body to below terminal CBD. 5/7 for rest of the area.
IMAGE REVIEW	:
POST PROCESSING	
• Recon algorithm/FOV	: STD/35 mm depending on patient size.
• Filter/Motion correction	: STD/Yes
• MPR/3D	: Nil/Nil
PHOTOGRAPHY	
• Window settings	: 350/50
• Printing format	: 17 × 14 –12 on 1 film for plain series
	: 17 × 14 –16 on 2 film for contrast series

CCT-RENAL SYSTEM

INDICATIONS	: Trauma, acute pyelonephritis, haematuria evaluation, renal or vesical mass, retroperitoneal masses
ENHANCEMENT TECHNIQUES	
• Oral	: 1500 ml of 1.5-2% diluted contrast media may be given orally at a rate of 200 ml/15 minutes before the scan
• Rectal	: 500 ml of 2% diluted contrast media may be given in all cases suspected to have pelvic or large bowel pathology.
• IV-ml/ Delay	: 100 ml/scan immediately after injection

PATIENT POSITIONING : Head first, Supine

PATENT INSTRUCTIONS : Patient is instructed to hold the breath.

SCANOGRAM : Abdomen AP.

REFERANCE LINE : Xiphisternum

SCAN REGION : Dome of diaphragm to pubic symphysis.

SCAN PLANE : Axial

SCAN PARAMETERS

- Algorithm/ kV/mA : STD/120 kV/140 mA
- SFOV/Time : 45/2 sec
- Slice thickness : Precontrast10/15 from dome of diaphragm to pubic symphysis. 10/10 from dome of diaphragm to top of kidneys. 5/7 from top of kidneys to lower pole of kidney. 10/10 lower pole of kidney to upper boarder of bladder. 5/7 for pelvis. Delayed scan may be required for contrast filled pelvicalyceal system and bladder

SPECIAL INSTRUCTIONS : Keep the urinay bladder full during scanning. Clamp the foley's catheter if catheterized.

IMAGE REVIEW :

POST PROCESSING

- Recon algorithm/ FOV : STD/35 mm depending on patient size.
- Filter/Motion correction : STD/Yes
- MPR/3D : Coronal and sagittal /Nil

PHOTOGRAPHY

- Window settings : 350/50
- Printing format : 17 × 14 – 12 on 1 film for plain series
  : 17 × 14 – 16 on 2 film for contrast series

CCT-ADRENAL GLAND

INDICATIONS : Neoplasm, infection, hyperplasia

ENHANCEMENT TECHNIQUES

- Oral : 500 ml of 1.5-2% diluted contrast media may be given orally at a rate of 100 ml/10 minutes before the scan
- Rectal : NIL.
- IV-ml/ Delay : 50 ml/scan immediately after injection

PATIENT POSITIONING : Head first, Supine
- Scan plane : Axial.

PATIENT INSTRUCTIONS : Patient is instructed to hold the breath.

SCANOGRAM : Abdomen AP.

REFERENCE LINE : Xiphisternum.

SCAN REGION : Tip of xyphoid to L-3 level

SCAN PLANE : Axial

SCAN PARAMETERS
- Algorithm/ Kv/mA : STD/120 kV/140 mA
- SFOV/Time : 45 cm/2 sec
- Slice thickness : 10/10 pre-contrast, T12 to L-2 level, 3/3 to cover the adrenal gland.

SPECIAL INSTRUCTIONS : The scan volume may be increased according to the extent of the mass. IV contrast should be used with caution in phaeochromocytoma.

IMAGE REVIEW : In clinically suspected phaeochromocytoma, if no adrenal mass is seen, the entire abdomen and pelvis should be screened for paraganglioma.

POST PROCESSING
- Recon algorithm/FOV : STD/35 cm depending on patient size. Targetted reconstruction with an FOV just to encompass the adrenal gland may be done
- Filter/ Motion correction : STD/Yes
- MPR/3D : Coronal and sagittal/Nil

PHOTOGRAPHY
- Window settings : 350/50
- Printing format : 17 × 14 –12 on 1 film for plain series
  : 17 × 14 –16 on 1 film for contrast series

CCT-PELVIS

INDICATIONS : Ca cervix, bladder, rectum, prostate, inflammation, trauma.

ENHANCEMENT TECHNIQUES
- Oral : 750 ml of 1.5-2% diluted contrast media may be given orally at a rate of 100 ml/10 minutes before the scan

• Rectal	: 500 ml.
• Vaginal	: Vagina may be packed with cotton/gauze soaked in diluted contrast media.
• IV-ml/ Delay	: 50 ml/scan immediately after injection
PATIENT POSITIONING	: Head first, Supine
PATIENT INSTRUCTIONS	: Patient is instructed to hold the breath.
SCANOGRAM	: Abdomen AP.
REFERENCE LINE	: Xiphisternum
SCAN REGION	: Iliac crest to pubic symphysis.
SCAN PLANE	: Axial
SCAN PARAMETERS	
• Algorithm/ kV/mA	: STD/120 kV/140 mA
• SFOV/Time	: 35/2 sec
• Slice thickness	: 10/10 pre-contrast from iliac crest to pubic symphysis. Post-contrast 55
SPECIAL INSTRUCTIONS	: Colonic preparation and air contrast is required for staging of rectal ca. Urinary bladder should be kept full during the scan (clamp the catheter if present). Delayed scan after contrast opacification of bladder may be require as the situation demands (bladder tumour, VVF, RVF etc)
IMAGE REVIEW	: Additional scan for abdomen proper may be required depending on the findings
POST PROCESSING	
• Recon algorithm/FOV	: STD/35 cm depending on patient size. Targetted reconstruction with an FOV just to encompass the adrenal gland may be done
• Filter/ Motion correction	: STD/Yes
• MPR/3D	: Coronal and sagittal /Nil
PHOTOGRAPHY	
• Window settings	: 350/50
• Printing format	: 17 × 14 –12 on 1 film for plain series.

PROTOCOLS PROTOCOLS FOR CT SPINE AND MUSCULO SKELETAL SYSTEM

SPINE

The neck is moderately flexed to reduce the normal cervical lordosis so as to make the axial sections nearly parallel to the disc spaces for cervical spine.

For the study of the L4-L5 and L5-S1 discs, the gantry tilt may not be adequate enough for the axial scan and so flexion of hips and knees supported by the pillow may be needed to bring the plane of the lumbar disc within the range of the machine. Many radiologists prefer scanning en block and then use MPR through the plane of the individual disc of interest and study the sagittal paraaxial reconstructions are required

Extremities

The slice thickness and spacing depend on the body region and size and site of the lesion in question. The long bones and joints may need 10 mm or 5 mm slice. At times the entire affected bone may have to be scanned.

CCT-HIP

INDICATIONS : Trauma, osteonecrosis, tumour, infection, inflammation, trauma.

ENHANCEMENT TECHNIQUES

- Oral : NIL
- Rectal : NIL
- IV-ml/ Delay : NIL

PATIENT POSITIONING : Head first/Supine.

SCANOGRAM : Pelvis AP

SCAN REGION : Iliac crest to pubic symphysis

SCAN PLANE : Axial

SCAN PARAMETERS

- Algorithm/kV/mA : STD/120 kV/140 mA
- SFOV/Time : 35/2 sec
- Slice thickness : 10/10 from iliac crest to roof of acetabulum.
  : 3/3 from roof to inferior border of acetabulum. 10/10 from acetabular floor tip to ischial tuberosity

SPECIAL INSTRUCTIONS : If the patient is investigated for avascular necrosis 3/3 mm scan from roof to floor of acatabulum is good enough.

IMAGE REVIEW : Additional scan for abdomen proper may be required depending on the findings

POST PROCESSING

- Recon algorithm/FOV : Bone/35 cm depending on patient size. Targetted reconstruction with an FOV just to encompass individual hip joints separately may be useful

- Filter/Motion correction : Sharp/Yes
- MPR/3D : Coronal and sagittal/If possible especially in trauma

PHOTOGRAPHY
- Window settings : 2000/750
- Printing format : 17 × 14 –16 on 1 film for plain series

CCT–SI JOINTS

INDICATIONS : Sacroiliac arthritis

ENHANCEMENT TECHNIQUES
- Oral : Nil
- Rectal : Nil
- IV-ml/Delay : Nil

PATIENT POSITIONING : Head first/Supine with knee flexed slightly

SCANOGRAM : AP Pelvis. Table postion adjusted so that sacrum is in the centre.

SCAN REGION : S1 vertebrae to lower SI joint.

SCAN PLANE : Axial with 20 degree forward angulation

SCAN PARAMETERS
- Algorithm/ kV/mA : Bone/120 kV/140 mA
- SFOV/Time : 35/3 sec
- Slice thickness : 2/5 mm

IMAGE REVIEW :

POST PROCESSING
- Recon algorithm/FOV : Bone/20 depending on patient size.
- Filter/Motion correction : Sharp/Yes
- MPR/3D : Nil/Nil

PHOTOGRAPHY
- Window settings : 350/50
- Printing format : 17 × 14 –12 on 1 film for plain series
  : 17 x 14 –16 on 1 film for contrast series

CHAPTER 13

Spiral CT

I. INTRODUCTION

Spiral (helical) or volume CT is a technique where by the patient is transported continuously through the gantry while data are acquired continuously during several 360^0 scans. The technique is so named because the x-ray can be thought of as tracing a helix or spiral curve on the patient's surface. Each rotation of x-ray tube can be thought of as generating data specific to an angled plane of section. Transaxial image may be reconstructed only after a full complement of data specific to each plane of section is estimated. The mathematical estimation is performed by interpolation. This computer software adjusts for the slight angle by arranging the data and creating an image that is not slanted.

II. REQUIREMENTS FOR VOLUME DATA ACQUISITION

1. Continuously rotating scanner based on slip-ring technology.
2. Continuous couch movement.
3. Increased loadability of the x-ray tube, capable of delivering at least 200 mA per revolution continuously throughout the time it takes to scan the volume of tissue (in addition, an increase in cooling capability is required compared to that in a nonspiral system).
4. Spiral-helical weighting algorithm.
5. Mass memory buffer to store the vast amount of data collected.

III. ADVANCES OF SPIRAL SCANNER OVER CONVENTIONAL CT

1. Slip ring device.
2. More efficient tube cooling.

3. Increased milliampere capability.
4. Smoother table movement.
5. Software adjusting for table movement.
6. Efficient detectors.

IV. HARDWARE CONSIDERATIONS

SLIP-RING TECHNOLOGY

Basic concepts

The need for faster scan times and for improvements in three-dimensional and multi-planar reconstruction has encouraged the development of continuous rotation scanners, in which the data is collected in volumes rather than slice-by-slice. In spiral CT system the gantry rotates continually in the same direction. In contrast, the conventional system which makes a 360° rotation in one direction, comes to a complete stop, then turns 360° in the opposing direction. Spiral–helical CT is made possible through the use of slip–ring technology, which allows for continuous gantry rotation. Slip-rings are "electromechanical devices consisting of circular electrical conductive rings and brushes that transmit electrical energy across a rotating interface". The slip-ring tube is also referred to as a continuous rotation gantry. Because the gantry does not require continuous stopping and starting, it can reach a much higher rotational speed within the gantry. Consequently this higher rotational speed accounts for the reduced scan time. To maintain the same quality image, the milliampere setting must be increased when scan time is decreased.

The development of quicker, smoother moving tables was essential in reducing the time between axial scans. Improving table features was vital in the development of continuous acquisition. With slip-ring technology there is no electrical cable connecting the gantry components to the ground and the source detector assembly will rotate voltage for control systems continuously. There are multiple parallel slip rings with one supplying high voltage to the tube and generator, one exchanging digital data between the computer and source detector assembly and a third providing low voltage for control systems.

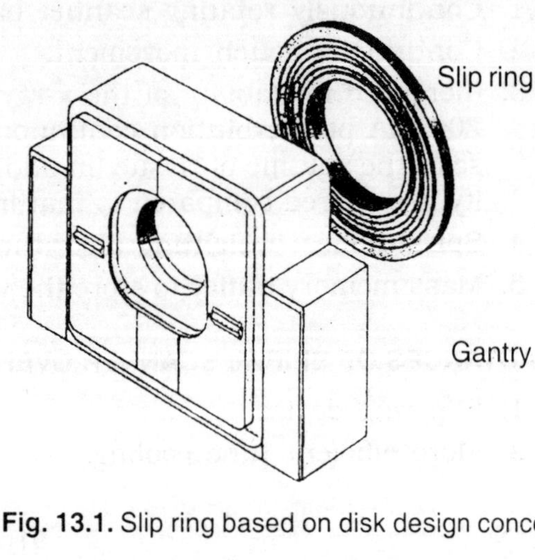

Fig. 13.1. Slip ring based on disk design concept.

The conventional CT machine had a delay of 3.5 sec after each exposure. This was for unwinding the tube for 360° rotation. Slip-ring technology basically abolishes the need for cables between generator and anode. Instead power from generator is connected to a large stationary ring made of suitable conductor. Another large ring which houses the x-ray tube and detectors moves around the stationary ring. Power is transmitted from stationary ring to the anode by means of brushes.

Design and Power Supply of Slip Rings

There are two types of slip-ring designs for use in CT scanners, the disk and the cylinder. The conductive rings are positioned so that they form concentric circles that lie in the plane of rotation. The cylindric design, on the other hand, has the conductive rings positioned (along the axis of rotation) so that they form a cylinder. The brushes that transmit electrical power to the CT components glide in contact grooves on the stationary slip ring. Two types of brush design are commonly used, the wire brush and the composite brush. The wire brush uses conductive wire as a sliding contact. "A brush consists of one or more wires arranged such that they function as a cantilever spring with a free end against the conductive ring. Two brushes per ring are often used to increase either communication reliability or current carrying capacity. The composite brush uses a block of some conductive material (e.g. a sliver–graphite alloy) as a sliding contact. Slip-ring scanners are intended to provide continuous rotation of the gantry by eliminating the long, high-tension cables to the x-ray tube used in conventional start-stop scanners, which must be unwound after a complete rotation. Slip-ring scanners have their high-voltage generators located in the gantry. Based on the power supply to the slip ring, which in turn provides power to the CT components in the gantry. Two categories of slip-ring scanners are available, scanners with low-voltage or high-voltage slip rings.

Milliampere-Second and Tube Cooling Limitations

The scan time options are limited; it is sometimes difficult to maintain an appropriate milliampere-second level. If this level is not maintained, quantum noise results, as in axial images. Continuous x-ray production generates a tremendous amount of heat. However, to scan for such long periods and consequently cover more anatomy per scan, the milliampere setting must be lowered. The technologist must maintain the setting above the minimum exposure necessary to produce a satisfactory image. Like cluster scanning, some systems allow the technologist to break spiral scans into groups to allow the patient to breathe. This practice also allows some time for the tube to cool so that higher milliampere settings can be used.

V. SOFT WARE CONSIDERATION

Interpolation algorithm is the mathematical process by which missing data are estimated in helical CT data sets. In the initial helical CT scans missing data were generated by linear interpolation using data points separated by a full 360 degree rotation of X-ray (360 degree interpolation). The axial images reconstructed from such data were nearly identical to conventional scanning. Blurring was a serious problem in longitudinal reformations along the direction of table travel (Z axis). A new interpolation algorithm that improved longitudinal resolution by using data closer to the desired plane of section was developed. This 180 degree interpolation increased longitudinal resolution at the expense of increased noise. The advantages of 180 degree interpolation over 360 interpolation are:

1. Higher pitch can be used (more than 1:1)
2. Reduced effective slice thickness
3. Better longitudinal resolution

VI. PROCEDURE OF SPIRAL ACQUISITION

Basic Spiral Scan Procedure

Spiral scanning is accomplished in the same way as axial slice:

(1) A scout image is obtained.
(2) The location of the spiral images are determined from the scout image.
(3) The patient is asked to hold his/her breath (for body studies).
(4) Data are acquired in varying amounts, depending on the type of scan.
(5) The patient is allowed to breath.
(6) Steps 3-5 through are repeated until all areas of interest are covered.
(7) The data are reconstructed into images that are displayed on the monitor.

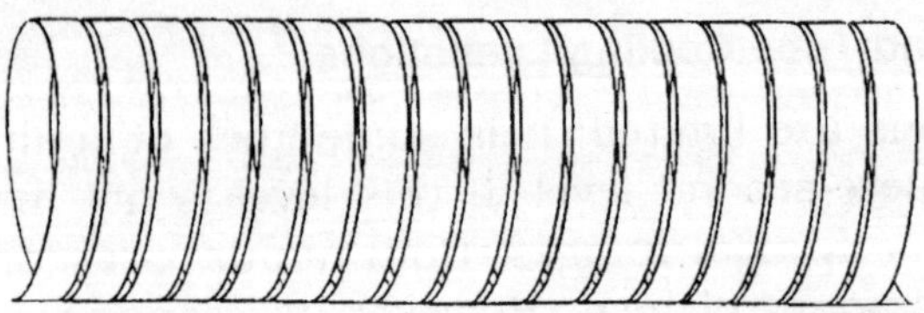

Fig. 11.2. Spiral scan gives slices at a slight angulation

Pitch

The relation of table speed to slice thickness is referred to as pitch. If the slice thickness is set at 5 mm, the table moves at a speed that allows the gantry to rotate once every 5 mm of table travel. If the pitch is adjusted to 2 : 1 and the

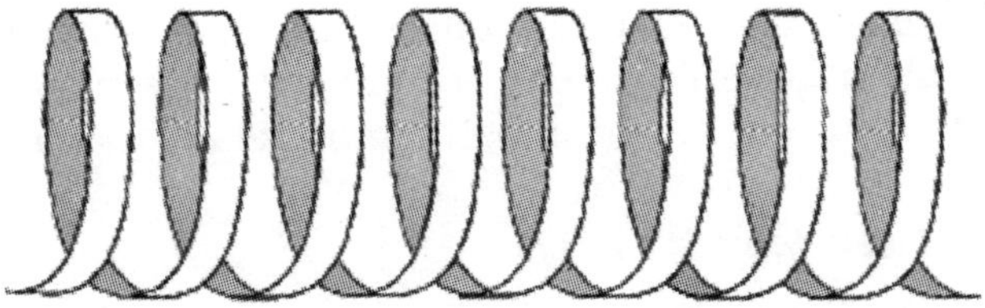

Fig. 11.3. Effects of increasing pitch

slice thickness is maintained at 5 mm, the tube rotates only once for every 10 mm of table motion. This procedure is similar to stretching a spring.

Increasing pitch increases the effective slice thickness because more information must be interpolated to produce an image. Increasing effective slice thickness decreases image resolution. Pitch is directly proportional to effective slice thickness as well as resolution. Increasing pitch is sometimes used to speed scanning for pediatric patients or patients with acute trauma. Pitch may also be increased when covering a longer anatomic area in the shortest time possible is of paramount importance, such as the case in CT angiography. Another rationale for increasing pitch is to cover more data in each patient breath hold, thereby reducing slice misregistration. Increasing the pitch will reduce total radiation dose to the patient. On some scanners, it is possible to decrease pitch to less than 1:1. In such cases, the table moves more slowly so that the data are actually overlapping, with some areas of anatomy being exposed twice.

$$\text{Pitch} = \frac{\text{Table feed} \times \text{time per rotation of 360}}{\text{Collimation}}$$

$$\text{Simply, Pitch} = \frac{\text{Table feed}}{\text{Collimation}}, \text{ if it is a 1 Second scan}$$

Collimation and Table feed

For example Table feed 5 mm, Collimation 5 mm, Pitch = 1 : 1
Table feed 7.5 mm, Collimation 5 mm, Pitch = 1.5 : 1
Table feed 10 mm, Collimation 5 mm, Pitch = 2 : 1

Area coverage

5 mm thickness 30 sec scan

1. Pitch 1 : 1 = 15 cm
2. Pitch 1.5 : 1 = 22.5 cm
3. Pitch 2 : 1 = 30 cm

As the pitch is higher, resolution is poor. Since the effective slice thickness increase, 30% increase in slice thickness is expected with a 2 : 1 pitch.

In most cases, scanning with thinner collimation at a higher pitch value produces a smaller effective slice thickness than with the next selectable collimation value and a pitch of 1:1 on most commercially available scanners.

Scan formula for a 1 sec scan 1:1 Pitch

$$\text{No. of images} = \frac{\text{Acquisition time}}{\text{Single rotation time}}$$

Area covered = No. of images × slice thickness

Reconstruction (retrospective changing of slice incrementation)

An advantage of spiral scanning is the ability to change the reconstructed slice incrementation. Because the data are acquired continually, raw data can be reconstructed retrospectively at any point. In this way, staggered slices can be created with as little as 1 mm difference. The goal of this approach is to show the abnormality on only one image. Because this method reduces the normal tissue that is averaged in, the measurement is more accurate. These reconstructions can be staggered by as little as 1 mm; in this way, an additional 90 images can be created from the same 10 seconds data. Creating a series of overlapping images produces superior three-dimensional and multiplanar reformatted images and can be done without increased radiation exposure to the patient. Although the slice incrementation can be changed with the raw data, it is impossible to change the actual slice thickness because the data are obtained in ribbons, and not as a block at a time. Slice thickness is controlled by the physical opening of the collimator and cannot be changed retrospectively. The only way to obtain a thinner slice is to rescan the area.

Longitudinal resolution is lesser than conventional scanning because of broadening of slice profile with helical aquisition. Degree of slice broadening is proportional to table feed. The reconstruction interval may be retrospectively and arbitrarily chosen after helical acquisition to produce images separated by no more than 1 mm. When the reconstruction interval exceeds the collimation longitudinal resolution is equal to the reconstruction interval. For reconstruction intervals less than the collimation, longitudinal resolution improves to a certain plateau. This plateau occurs at 20% overlap if pitch is 2 : 1 and at 40% overlap if pitch is 1 : 1. Hence reconstruction interval with >50% overlap will not provide any substantial benefit.

Effective slice thickness

The slice beginning does not match the slice end, each rotation is at a slight angle. Computer software adjusts for this slight angle by averaging the data and creating an image that is not slanted. This software process is referred to as interpolation and is a complex statistical method of processing data.

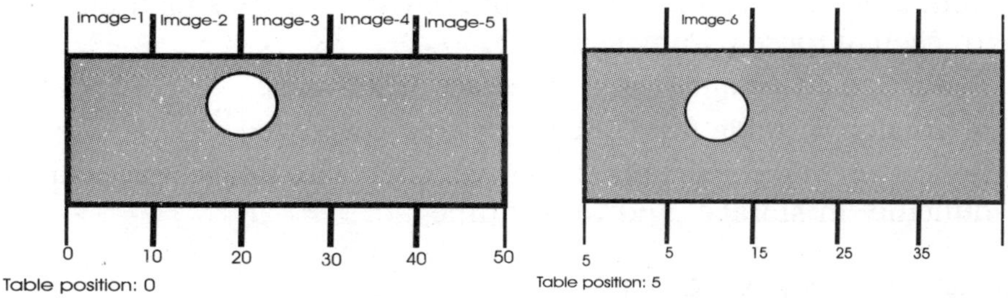

Fig. 11.3. Reducing partial volume effect by changing the incrementation of spiral data retrospectively.

Different interpolation formulas are used and have varying degrees of accuracy. Because of this software interpolation, the effective slice thickness is greater than the collimator opening. The degree to which the slice thickness is enlarged is dependent on the efficiency of the software. The effect is negligible when a pitch of 1 : 1 is used. To summarize, slice thickness is affected to varying degrees and is dependent on pitch selection, selected slice thickness and manufacturer. However, no system eliminates this problem inherent in continuous acquisition scanning. Any interpolation causes a slight decrease in image resolution and a resulting loss of detail. In reality, this effect is minimal and is more than offset by the benefits of scanning at peak contrast enhancement. In most cases, an axial image and a spiral image appear identical.

VII. ARTIFACTS

1) Break up artifact

It is seen as an irregular disruption of a transverse high contrast interface on longitudinal reformations. This artifact is usually seen with 180 degree nonlinear interpolations. It is not seen with 360 linear or 180 degree linear interpolations.

2) Stair step artifact

This artifact also is unique to helical CT. It is seen as high contrast interfaces in longitudinal reformation and manifest as disruption of inclined surfaces in a regular stair step fashion. The height of the step longitudinally is proportional to table feed and independent of collimation or reconstruction interval. This artifact is independent of interpolation used also. It is most apparent with narrow structures of high contrast that are imaged with zoom.

VIII. OPTIMIZING HELICAL CT

Care should be taken to maximize longitudinal resolution by minimizing collimation, table feed, reconstruction interval and recognising trade offs that exist with each of these parameters i.e. :

1. Reduction in collimation : Increases pixel noise
2. Reduction in table feed : Reduces area coverage
3. Reduction in reconstruction interval : Increases image processing time, difficulty in storage, and review time

IX. ADVANTAGES OF HELICAL CT

1. Increased speed of a study.
2. Exact continuity of images.
3. Less slice misregistration
4. Less motion artifact
5. Need for less contrast medium.
6. Different phase of vascular enhancement can be studied with single injection (dual/triple phase study)
7. Availability of volumetric data
   (a) Ability for retrospective reconstruction (ability to change slice incrimentation retrospectively)
   (b) Better 3D and reformatted images .

X. LIMITATIONS OF HELICAL CT

1. Requires very cooperative patient.
2. Reduction in image quality.
3. Requires precise timing of enhancement.
4. Costly machine and X-ray tube.
5. Slightly thicker slices than selected when pitch is greater than 1:1.
6. Loss of image resolution because of the interpolation required to process the spiral data.
7. Increased image noise if the milliampere settings cannot be maintained because of the tube limitations.

CHAPTER 14

Introduction to Spiral CT Technique and Protocols

The patient positioning is more or less same as for conventional CT. After the patient is positioned and scanogram is obtained the following steps can be used to plan a spiral CT.

1. Select slice thickness for the region of interest.
2. Pitch ratio is determined, depending upon the area to be covered. Larger pitch gives larger volume coverage with increased effective thickness of the sections. Smaller pitch ratio gives better image resolution and lower area coverage.
3. Area of scanning depending upon the table feed and scan time.
4. Since the patient cannot hold breath longer area coverage may require more than one series with a breath time in between. This may not be true with scans where breath holding is not necessary. But the tube limitations do not allow larger area coverage in one series.
5. Images are reconstructed using interpolation algorithms to rectify slanting effect of spiral CT.
6. Slice incrementation can be reduced during retrospective reconstruction.
7. It is always better to use pressure injector for contrast injection to cope up with the speed of helical scan. The amount and time delay varies from region to region depending upon the time taken for the contrast to flow from injection site to the organ concerned and the phase of flow we are interested. The amount of contrast required in spiral CT is lower than that would be required in conventional scan to provide the same amount of contrast enhancement. In the following description of spiral CT protocol it is assumed that all spiral CT scans use pressure injector and contrast technique description will be based on that.

8. One important technical limitation that should be remembered is that low-end spiral machines are usually provided with lower mA capability. Scan time may have to be increased to avoid grainy images.

THE ROLE OF SPIRAL CT IN HEAD AND NECK

Even if spiral CT facility is available most of the head scans are done as conventional axial sections. Remember the axial scan sections have more resolution than slanted spiral sections. Unless very essential spiral scans should not be done routinely for brain. The spiral scan of head is useful in the following situations

1. When a CT angiography is planned.
2. 3D CT is needed for craniofacial trauma.
3. Craniostenosis for 3D CT.
4. As a last resort in very restless patient and uncooperative children helical CT may be done for brain.

SCT-BRAIN PLAIN

INDICATIONS	: Uncooperative patient
ENHANCEMENT TECHNIQUES	
• Oral	: Nil
• IV-ml/Delay	: Nil
PATIENT POSITIONING	: Head First/Supine
PATIENT INSTRUCTIONS	: Nil
SCANOGRAM	: Skull lateral upto C_3
REFERENCE LINE	: Parallel to OM line
SCAN REGION	: Base of skull to vertex
SCAN PLANE	: Axial
SCAN PARAMETERS	
• Algorithm/kV/mA	: STD/140 kV/120 mA
• SFOV/Time	: 25 cm/1-2 sec
• Slice thickness	: 5 mm
• Table feed	: 7 mm
IMAGE REVIEW	: Look for small lesions and obtain thin section in the concerned region.
POST PROCESSING	
• Recon mode/FOV	: STD/19 cm
• Filter	: STD
• Reformation/3D	: Nil/Nil

PHOTOGRAPHY

- Window settings : 120/40 for post. fossa
  : 100/35 for supratentorial
- Printing format : 17 × 14 -12 on 1

SPECIAL NOTE : mAs can be reduced when small children and infants are studied

SCT–BRAIN FOR HEAD INJURY

INDICATIONS : Very uncooperative patient and when 3D reformation considered to be essential

ENHANCEMENT TECHNIQUES

- Oral : Nil
- IV-ml/Delay : Nil

PATIENT POSITIONING : Head First/Supine

PATIENT INSTRUCTIONS : Nil

SCANOGRAM : Skull lateral upto C3

REFERENCE LINE : Parallel to OM line

SCAN REGION : Base of skull to vertex

SCAN PLANE : Axial

SCAN PARAMETERS

- Algorithm/kV/mA : STD/140 kV/120 mA
- SFOV/Time : 25 cm/1-2 sec
- Slice thickness : 5 mm
- Table feed : 7 mm

IMAGE REVIEW :

POST PROCESSING

- Recon mode/FOV : STD and bone/19 cm
  Additional reconstructed in soft algorithm at 2.5 mm increment is done when 3D imaging is considered.
- Filter : Sharp for bone
- Reformation/3D : Done

PHOTOGRAPHY

- Window settings : 120/40 for post. fossa
  : 100/35 for supratentorial
- Printing format : 17 × 14 -12 on 1

SCT-FOR FACIAL TRAUMA

INDICATIONS	: Extensive facial trauma where reconstructive plastic surgery would be required. Clinician is particular about 3D
ENHANCEMENT TECHNIQUES	
• Oral	: Nil
• IV-ml/Delay	: Nil
PATIENT POSITIONING	: Head First/Supine
PATIENT INSTRUCTIONS	: Nil
SCANOGRAM	: Skull lateral up to C3
REFERENCE LINE	: Parallel to OM line
SCAN REGION	: Supraorbital ridge to below symphysis menti or the area specified by the surgeon
SCAN PLANE	: Axial
SCAN PARAMETERS	
• Algorithm/kV/mA/	: STD/140 kV/120 mA
• SFOV/Time	: 25 cm - 1-2 sec
• Slice thickness	: 3 mm
• Table feed	: 5 mm
IMAGE REVIEW	:
POST PROCESSING	
• Recon mode/FOV	: STD and bone/19 cm. Additional reconstruction in soft algorithm at 1.5 mm increment is done for 3D reformation considered.
• Filter	: Sharp for bone
• Reformation/3D	: Done in SSD
PHOTOGRAPHY	
• Window settings	: 120/40 for post fossa
	: 100/35 for supratentorial
• Printing format	: 17 × 14 -12 on 1

SCT–CORONAL SINUS CT

INDICATIONS	: Sinusitis, trauma, tumour, polyps.
ENHANCEMENT TECHNIQUES	
• Oral	: Nil
• IV-ml/ Delay	: Nil
PATIENT POSITIONING	: Head first/Prone

PATIENT INSTRUCTIONS	:
SCANOGRAM	: Skull lateral
REFERENCE LINE	: Perpendicular to hard palate
SCAN REGION	: From anterior nasal bone to post sphenoid sinus.
SCAN PLANE	: Coronal
SCAN PARAMETERS	
• Algorithm/kV/mA	: STD/140 kV/140 mA
• SFOV/Time	: 25/2 sec
• Slice thickness/Time	: 5/5 mm
SPECIAL INSTRUCTIONS	: Contrast may be useful in tumour cases
IMAGE REVIEW	: Nil
POST PROCESSING	
• Recon algorithm/FOV	: Bone/15 cm
• Filter/Motion correction	: Sharp/Nil
• Reformation/3D	: Sagittal/may be done
PHOTOGRAPHY	
• Window settings	: 280/40 for soft tissue.
	: 3500/700 for bone window.
• Printing format	: 17 × 14 -16 on 1
SPECIAL NOTE	: This is the recommended plane of scan for orbital blowout fractures

SCT–NECK SURVEY

INDICATIONS	: Lymph node screening.
ENHANCEMENT TECHNIQUES	
• Oral	: Nil
• IV-ml/Delay	: 50 ml/2 ml/sec/30 sec delay
PATIENT POSITIONING	: Head first/Supine
PATIENT INSTRUCTIONS	: Nil
SCANOGRAM	: Neck lateral
REFERENCE LINE	: Parallel to vertebral end plate
SCAN REGION	: Base of skull to thoracic inlet
SCAN PLANE	: Axial
SCAN PARAMETERS	
• Algorithm/ kV/mA	: STD/120 kV/140 mA
• SFOV/Time	: 25 cm/2 sec
• Slice thickness	: 5 mm
• Table feed	: 7 mm

SPECIAL INSTRUCTIONS : Gantry angulation appropriate to exclude dental artifacts.

IMAGE REVIEW : Nil

POST PROCESSING

- Recon algorithm/FOV : STD/Just to fit neck
- Filter/Motion correction : STD/ Yes.
- MPR/3D : Coronal/Nil

PHOTOGRAPHY

- Window settings : 240/40 soft tissue.
- Printing format : 17 × 14 -16 on 1

SCT–PHARYNX

INDICATIONS : Neoplasm, inflammation

ENHANCEMENT TECHNIQUES

- Oral : Nil
- IV-ml/Delay : 50 ml/2 ml/sec/30 sec delay

PATIENT POSITIONING : Head first/Supine

PATIENT INSTRUCTIONS : Patient is instructed not to swallow during scanning

SCANOGRAM : Neck lateral

REFERENCE LINE : Parallel to vertebral end plate

SCAN REGION : Base of skull to hyoid bone

SCAN PLANE : Axial. Coronal study is useful in nasopharynx

SCAN PARAMETERS

- Algorithm/kV/mA : STD/120 kV/140 mA
- SFOV/Time : 25/2 sec
- Slice thickness : 5/7 mm

SPECIAL INSTRUCTIONS : Appropriate gantry angulation to exclude dental artifacts

IMAGE REVIEW : Nil

POST PROCESSING

- Recon algorithm/FOV : STD/Include neck in case of cervical adenopathy
- Filter/Motion correction : STD/If needed
- MPR/3D : Sagittal and coronal/Nil

PHOTOGRAPHY

- Window settings : 240/40
- Printing format : 17 × 14 -16 on 1

SCT–LARYNX

INDICATIONS	: Neoplasm, inflammation. Cong lesions.
ENHANCEMENT TECHNIQUES	
• Oral	: Nil
• IV-ml/ Delay	: 50 ml/2 ml/sec/30 sec delay
PATIENT POSITIONING	: Head first, supine
PATIENT INSTRUCTIONS	: Patient is instructed not to swallow during scanning
SCANOGRAM	: Neck lateral.
REFERENCE LINE	: Parallel to vertebral endplate
SCAN REGION	: Epiglottis to below cricoid cartilage.
SCAN PLANE	: Axial
SCAN PARAMETERS	
• Algorithm/kV/mA	: STD/120 kV/140 mA
• SFOV/Time	: 25/2 sec
• Slice thickness	: 3/5 mm. Additional 1 mm sections may be obtained for vocal cord
SPECIAL INSTRUCTIONS	: Valsalva manoeuvre and phonation are useful for airway evaluation. Patient is instructed not to swallow and breathe.
IMAGE REVIEW	: Nil
POST PROCESSING	
• Recon algorithm/FOV	: STD/15 cm
• Filter/Motion correction	: STD/If needed
• MPR/3D	: Sagittal and coronal/Nil
PHOTOGRAPHY	
• Window settings	: 240/40
• Printing format	: 17 × 14 -16 on 1

PROTOCOLS FOR SCT CHEST

BENEFITS OF SCT

1. The major benefit here is elimination of respiratory movement misregistration in SCT
2. Artifacts caused on CCT while evaluating lung bases due to diaphragmatic motion are eliminated in SCT.
3. Pulmonary nodules though very small are better delineated in SCT by employing slice-shifting technique.

4. SCT allows fast and vivid MPR and 3D reconstructions, which are helpful in demonstrating tracheal tumours, other tracheal lesions, bronchial dehiscence, and also in evaluating thoracic vasculature aortic, aneurysms and dissections.
5. As volume data can be useful for reconstruction of the thinner image slices, SCT is exclusively special in the areas of suspected airway pathology.
6. Smaller amounts of contrast medium are sufficient for rapid CT study in thoracic evaluation as compared to CCT (60 ml against 200 ml).
7. Peak contrast opacification facilitates detection of a central/segmental pulmonary emboli/vascular anomaly/AVM's with ease.

SCT–CHEST PLAIN SCREENING

INDICATIONS	: Screening for subtle neoplasm or inflammation
ENHANCEMENT TECHNIQUES	
• Oral	: Nil
• IV-ml/ Delay	: NIl
PATIENT POSITIONING	: Head first, supine
PATIENT INSTRUCTIONS	: Patient is instructed to hold the breath in full inspiration and to keep the level of inspiration same at all sections
SCANOGRAM	: Chest AP
SCAN REGION	: Apex to lung base
REFERENCE LINE	: Sternal notch
SCAN PLANE	: Axial
SCAN PARAMETERS	
• Algorithm/ kV/mA	: STD/120 kV/160 mA
• SFOV/Time	: 35/1-2 sec
• Slice thickness	: 10/10
SPECIAL INSTRUCTIONS	: If mediastinal or lung masses are visualized contrast study may be required
POST PROCESSING	
• Recon algorithm/FOV	: Sharp/30 cm depending on patient size
• Filter/Motion correction	: Lung/If needed
• MPR/3D	: Nil/Nil
PHOTOGRAPHY	
• Window settings	: 1500/700 for lungs
	: 350/50 for mediastinum

• Printing format	: 17 × 14 -16 on 1 for lungs
	: 17 × 14 -16 on 1 for mediastinum

SCT–CHEST FOR MASS LESIONS

INDICATIONS	: Lung, mediastinal, pleural or esophageal mass lesions, inflammatory and congenital lesions, empyema, chest wall pathologies
ENHANCEMENT TECHNIQUES	
• Oral	: Nil
• IV-ml/ Delay	: 50 ml/3 ml/sec/30 sec delay.
PATIENT POSITIONING	: Head first, supine
PATIENT INSTRUCTIONS	: 4 hours fasting before the study
SCANOGRAM	: Chest AP.
REFERENCE LINE	: Sternal notch
SCAN REGION	: Lung apex to adrenal levels.
SCAN PLANE	: Axial
SCAN PARAMETERS	
• Algorithm/kV/mA	: STD/120 kV/160 mA
• SFOV/Time	: 35/1-2 sec
• Slice thickness	: 10/10 plain 10/10 from apex to 25 mm above carina. 5/5 from 25 mm above carina to 60 mm below carina. 10/10 from 60 mm below carina to adrenal level
SPECIAL INSTRUCTIONS	: Breath holding in deep inspiration and maintain the same level of inspiration at all slices should be advised and demonstrated. Oral contrast may be given in cases of esophageal pathology. Extend the study to the level of celiac axis in cases of esophageal malignancy. Additional prone scanning may be done in cases of fungal ball in a cavity.
POST PROCESSING	
• Recon algorithm FOV	: Sharp for lung /30 depending on patient size
• Filter/Motion correction	: Lung/If needed.
• MPR/3D	: Nil/Nil

PHOTOGRAPHY

- Window settings : 1500/700 for lungs. 350/50 mediastinum.
- Printing format : 17 × 14 -12 on 1 for lungs 2 films
  : 17 × 14 -16 on 1 for mediastinum

PROTOCOLS FOR CT ABDOMEN

Only for detection of or characterization for small masses, overlapping reconstructions are useful. For MPR 3D reconstruction very small IRI provide better detail. Nasogastric tube feed of contrast medium is to be resorted to when the patient cannot drink oral contrast medium. In patients having symptoms of bowel obstruction, contrast medium should be given the night before the scheduled scan, to get adequate bowel opacification. Delayed images during excretory phase distinguish parapelvic cyst from hydronephrosis. In RCC patient, arterial tumour vascularity and renal vein invasion are readily assessed. 3D imaging provides help for assessing renal artery stenosis. SCT also helps in detection of renal calculi (non-contrast CT)

CECT is performed for angiographic information about vascular structures and for gross cardiac anatomy and for distinguishing tumours from blood vessels (during biopsy), to estimate blood flow to a lesion of solid or cystic type.

Liver: Each study has to be planned individually after review of clinical problem and the capabilities of the scanner. The opacification of GIT with oral contrast is standard for all studies of CT abdomen.

Spleen: Spleen being a highly vascular organ, it has peak levels of contrast enhancement shortly after aorta. On CECT, spleen displays CT value of 100-150 HU during arterial phase and 60-100 HU in venous phase.

SCT–WHOLE ABDOMINAL AND PELVIS SCREENING

INDICATIONS : Screening for neoplasm, infective foci,

ENHANCEMENT TECHNIQUES

- Oral : 1500 ml of 1.5-2% diluted contrast media may be given orally at a rate of 200 ml/15 minutes before the scan
- Rectal : 500 ml of 2% diluted contrast media may be given in all cases suspected to have pelvic or large bowel pathology.
- IV-ml/ Delay : May be used if there is any relevant positive findings on plain CT. 100 ml/2 ml/sec/40 sec delay.

PATIENT POSITIONING : Head first, supine.

PATIENT INSTRUCTIONS : Absolute breath hold in mid-inspiration and to maintain the same level of breath on each instruction.

SCANOGRAM : Abdomen AP

REFERENCE LINE : Xiphisternum

SCAN REGION : Dome of diaphragm to pubic symphysis

SCAN PLANE : Axial

SCAN PARAMETERS

- Algorithm/ kV/mA : STD/120 kV/140 mA
- SFOV/DFOV : 45/35
- Slice thickness/Time : 10 mm /2 sec

SPECIAL INSTRUCTIONS : Cluster scan facility if available may be used with 3-4 scans per breath followed by 15 sec breath time. Advised to maintain the same level of inspiration in all slices to avoid slice misregistration.

IMAGE REVIEW : Look for any pathology and perform post IV contrast CT with thin sections (5 mm).

POST PROCESSING

- Recon algorithm/FOV : STD/35 depending on patient size.
- Filter/Motion correction : STD/Yes
- MPR/3D : Nil/Nil

PHOTOGRAPHY

- Window settings : 350/50
- Printing format : 17 × 14 –16 on 1-2 films

SCT–WHOLE ABDOMEN AND PELVIS P+C

INDICATIONS : Suspected primary, metastatic Ca, neoplasia of GIT/urogenital system, PUO, Trauma,

ENHANCEMENT TECHNIQUES

- Oral : 1500 ml of 1.5-2% diluted contrast media may be given orally at a rate of 200 ml/15 minutes before the scan
- Rectal : 500 ml of 2% diluted contrast media may be given in all cases suspected to have pelvic or large bowel pathology.
- IV-ml/Delay : 100 ml/2 ml/sec/40 sec delay

PATIENT POSITIONING : Head first, supine

PATIENT INSTRUCTIONS	: Absolute breath hold in mid-inspiration and to maintain the same level of breath on each instruction.
SCANOGRAM	: Abdomen AP
REFERENCE LINE	: Xiphisternum
SCAN REGION	: Dome of diaphragm to pubic symphysis
SCAN PLANE	: Axial
SCAN PARAMETERS	
• Algorithm/kV/mA	: STD/120 kV/140 mA
• SFOV/DFOV	: 45/35
• Slice thickness	: 10 mm/10 mm plain CT. 5/7 mm from dome of diaphragm to lower pole of kidneys. 10/10 from lower pole of kidneys to iliac crest. 5/7 from iliac crest to pubic symphysis.
• Time	: 2 sec
SPECIAL INSTRUCTIONS	: Cluster scan facility if available may be used with 3-4 scans per breath followed by 15 sec breath time. Advised to maintain the same level of inspiration in all slices to avoid slice misregistration.
IMAGE REVIEW	: Look for any pathology and perform post IV contrast CT with thin sections (5 mm).
POST PROCESSING	
• Recon algorithm/FOV	: STD/35 depending on patient size
• Filter/Motion correction	: STD/Yes
• MPR/3D	: Nil/Nil
PHOTOGRAPHY	
• Window settings	: 350/50
• Printing format	: 17 × 14 –16 on 1-2 films

SCT–UPPER ABDOMEN FOR HEPATOBILIARY SYSTEM. P+C

INDICATIONS	: Tumours and inflammation of liver, pancreas, stomach,
ENHANCEMENT TECHNIQUES	
• Oral	: 1000 ml of 1.5-2% diluted contrast media may be given orally at a rate of 200 ml/15 minutes before the scan
• Rectal	: Nil
• IV-ml/Delay	: 100 ml-3 ml/sec-40 sec delay.

PATIENT POSITIONING	: Head first, Supine
PATIENT INSTRUCTIONS	: Absolute breath hold in mid-inspiration and to maintain the same level of breath on each instruction.
SCANOGRAM	: Abdomen AP
REFERENCE POINT	: Xiphisternum
SCAN REGION	: Dome of diaphragm to iliac crest symphysis.
SCAN PLANE	: Axial
SCAN PARAMETERS	
• Algorithm/kV/mA	: STD/120 kV/140 mA
• SFOV/Time	: 45/2 sec
• Slice thickness	: 10 mm/10 mm plain CT: 5/7 from dome of diaphragm to lower pole of kidneys. 10/10 from lower pole of kidneys to iliac crest
SPECIAL INSTRUCTIONS	: Cluster scan facility if available may be used with 3-4 scans per breath followed by 15 sec breath time. Advised to maintain the same level of inspiration in all slices to avoid slice misregistration.
IMAGE REVIEW	: Look for any pathology. Additional special scanning for liver, pancreas or kidneys may be required. In that case follow the instructions given in the corresponding sections.
POST-PROCESSING	
• Recon algorithm/FOV	: STD. /35 depending on patient size.
• Filter/ Motion correction	: STD/Yes
• MPR/3D	: Nil/Nil
PHOTOGRAPHY	
• Window settings	: 350/50
• Printing format	: 17 × 14 –20 on 1 film for plain series
	: 17 × 14 –20 on 2 film for contrast series

SCT–DEDICATED STUDY FOR HEPATIC HEMANGIOMA

INDICATIONS	: Strong suspicion of hepatic hemangioma for confirmation.
ENHANCEMENT TECHNIQUES	
• Oral	: Nil

- Rectal : Nil
- IV-ml/ Delay : 100 ml/3 ml/sec

PATIENT POSITIONING : Head first, supine

PATIENT INSTRUCTIONS : Absolute breath hold in mid-inspiration and to maintain the same level of breath on each instruction.

SCANOGRAM : Abdomen AP

REFERENCE LINE : Xiphisternum

SCAN REGION : Dome of diaphragm to lower pole of liver.

SCAN PLANE : Axial

SCAN PARAMETERS

- Algorithm/kV/mA : STD/120 kV/140 mA
- SFOV/Time : 45/2 sec
- Slice thickness : 10 mm/10 mm plain CT. Additional post contrast single location non-incremental scans are done through the centre of the lesion at 30 sec, 45 sec, 1 m, 2 m, 3 m, 5 m, 10 m, 20 m

SPECIAL INSTRUCTIONS : This dedicated study is done only to confirm hemangioma when the clinical and sonological suspicion is very high. But when the clinical situation demands differentiation of hemangioma from other hepatic tumours it is better to perform 5/7 post contrast study followed by additional delayed scan through the centre of the lesion.

IMAGE REVIEW : Look for centripetal type of nodular contrast filling from the periphery gradually filling the entire lesion over a period which is diagnostic of hemangioma.

POST PROCESSING

- Recon algorithm/FOV : STD/35 depending on patient size.
- Filter/ Motion correction : STD/Yes
- MPR/3D : Nil/Nil

PHOTOGRAPHY

- Window settings : 350/50
- Printing format : 17 × 14 –20 on 1 film for plain series
  : 17 × 14 –20 on 2 film for contrast series

SCT–DUAL PHASE CT OF LIVER

INDICATIONS	: Hepatocellular carcinoma, adenoma, hypervascular liver metastasis, focal nodular hyperplasia, mass in cirrhotic liver
ENHANCEMENT TECHNIQUES	
• Oral	: 1000 ml of 1.5-2% diluted contrast media may be given orally at a rate of 200 ml/15 minutes before the scan
• Rectal	: Nil
• IV-ml/ Delay	: 100 ml 3 ml/sec, 20 sec delay (arterial phase). 50-60 sec delay (venous phase)
PATIENT POSITIONING	: Head first, supine
PATIENT INSTRUCTIONS	: Absolute breath hold in mid-inspiration and to maintain the same level of breath on each instruction.
SCANOGRAM	: Abdomen AP.
REFERENCE POINT	: Xiphisternum
SCAN REGION	: Dome of diaphragm to lower pole of liver
SCAN PLANE	: Axial
SCAN PARAMETERS	
• Algorithm/ kV/mA	: STD/120 kV/140 mA
• SFOV/Time	: 45/1 sec
• Slice thickness	: 10/10 pre contrast. 5/7 from dome of diaphragm to lower pole for arterial phase. 5/7 from lower pole of liver to dome of diaphragm for venous phase.
IMAGE REVIEW	:
POST PROCESSING	
• Recon algorithm/FOV	: STD with 3.5 mm increment/35 mm depending on patient size.
• Filter/Motion correction	: STD/Yes
• MPR/3D	: Nil/Nil
PHOTOGRAPHY	
• Window settings	: 350/50
• Printing format	: 17 × 14 –12 on 1 film for plain series
	: 17 × 14 –16 on 2 film for contrast series

SCT–UPPER ABDOMEN FOR PANCREAS

INDICATIONS : Acute and chronic pancreatitis, pancreatic tumours, periampullary ca, cholangio ca

ENHANCEMENT TECHNIQUES

- Oral : 1000 ml of 1.5-2% diluted contrast media may be given orally at a rate of 200 ml/15 minutes before the scan
- Rectal : Nil
- IV-ml/ Delay : 100 ml/2 ml/sec/40 sec delay.

PATIENT POSITIONING : Head first, supine

PATIENT INSTRUCTIONS : Absolute breath hold in mid-inspiration and to maintain the same level of breath on each instruction.

SCANOGRAM : Abdomen AP

REFERANCE LINE : Xiphisternum

SCAN REGION : Dome of diaphragm to lower pole of kidney

SCAN PLANE : Axial

SCAN PARAMETERS

- Algorithm/ kV/mA : STD/120 kV/140 mA
- SFOV/Time : 45/2 sec
- Slice thickness : 10/10 pre-contrast. 5/7 from dome of diaphragm to just above pancreatic body. 3/5 from just above pancreatic body to below terminal CBD. 5/7 for rest of the area.

IMAGE REVIEW :

POST PROCESSING

- Recon algorithm/FOV : STD/35 mm depending on patient size.
- Filter/ Motion correction : STD/Yes
- MPR/3D : Nil/Nil

PHOTOGRAPHY

- Window settings : 350/50
- Printing format : 17 × 14 –12 on 1 film for plain series
  : 17 × 14 –16 on 2 film for contrast series

SCT-RENAL SYSTEM

INDICATIONS : Trauma, acute pyelonephritis, hematuria evaluation, renal or vesical mass, retroperitoneal masses

ENHANCEMENT TECHNIQUES	
• Oral	: 1500 ml of 1.5-2% diluted contrast media may be given orally at a rate of 200 ml/15 minutes before the scan
• Rectal	: 500 ml of 2% diluted contrast media may be given in all cases suspected to have pelvic or large bowel pathology.
• IV-ml/Delay	: 100 ml/3 ml/sec/40 sec delay.
PATIENT POSITIONING	: Head first, supine
PATIENT INSTRUCTIONS	: Absolute breath hold in mid-inspiration and to maintain the same level of breath on each instruction.
SCANOGRAM	: Abdomen AP
REFERENCE LINE	: Xiphisternum
SCAN REGION	: Dome of diaphragm to pubic symphysis
SCAN PLANE	: Axial
SCAN PARAMETERS	
• Algorithm/kV/mA	: STD/120 kV/140 mA
• SFOV/Time	: 45/2 sec
• Slice thickness	: Pre contrast 10/15 from dome of diaphragm to pubic symphysis. 10/10 from dome of diaphragm to top of kidneys. 5/7 from top of kidneys to lower pole of kidney. 10/10 lower pole of kidney to upper border of bladder. 5/7 for pelvis. Delayed scan may be required for contrast filled pelvicalyceal system and bladder.
SPECIAL INSTRUCTIONS	: Keep the urinay bladder full during scanning. Clamp the Foley's catheter if catheterized.
IMAGE REVIEW	:
POST PROCESSING	
• Recon algorithm/ FOV	: STD/35 mm depending on patient size
• Filter/Motion correction	: STD/Yes
• MPR/3D	: Coronal and sagittal/Nil
PHOTOGRAPHY	
• Window settings	: 350/50
• Printing format	: 17 × 14 –12 on 1 film for plain series
	: 17 × 14 –16 on 2 film for contrast series

SPECIAL NOTE : The CT appearance of renal enhancement after intravenous administration can be categorized into four phases: vascular, cortical nephrographic, paranchymal nephrographic and excretory. Renal vascularity is evaluated during the vascular phase, approximately 10-15 seconds after beginning of intravenous contrast material administration. A hyper-attenuating cortical nephrogram with corticomedullary differentiation is obtained during the cortical nephrographic phase, generally 20-45 sec after contrast material injection. In this phase normal renal anatomy can be exquisitely charecterized. Scan obtained during the parenchymal nephrographic phase, generally 45 seconds to 2 minutes after contrast material administration, reveals homogenous, uniform increased attenuation of renal parenchyma. In the excretory phase, the contrast material starts to appear in the collecting system approximately 2-3 minutes after contrast material administration. The precise timing of the various phases depends on the acquisition technique. The amount of contrast material and rate of administration depends on the cardiac output and the integrity of renal vasculature. The exact timing of the scanning depends on what information we are more interested in.

SCT–ADRENAL GLAND

INDICATIONS : Neoplasm, infection, hyperplasia

ENHANCEMENT TECHNIQUES

- Oral : 500 ml of 1.5-2% diluted contrast media may be given orally at a rate of 100 ml/10 minutes before the scan
- Rectal : Nil
- IV-ml/ Delay : 50 ml/3 ml/sec/40 sec delay.

PATIENT POSITIONING : Head first, supine

- Scan plane : Axial

PATIENT INSTRUCTIONS	: Absolute breath hold in mid-inspiration and to maintain the same level of breath on each instruction.
SCANOGRAM	: Abdomen AP.
REFERENCE LINE	: Xyphisternum.
SCAN REGION	: Tip of xyphoid to L-3 level
SCAN PLANE	: Axial
SCAN PARAMETERS	
• Algorithm/ kV/mA	: STD/120 kV/140 mA
• SFOV/Time	: 45 cm/2 sec
• Slice thickness	: 10/10 pre-contrast, T12 to L-2 level
	: 3/3 to cover the adrenal gland
SPECIAL INSTRUCTIONS	: The scan volume may be increased according to the extent of the mass. IV contrast should be used with caution in phaeochromocytoma.
IMAGE REVIEW	: In clinically suspected phaeochromocytoma, if no adrenal mass is seen, the entire abdomen and pelvis should be screened for paraganglioma
POST PROCESSING	
• Recon algorithm/FOV	: STD/35 cm depending on patient size. Targetted reconstruction with an FOV just to encompass the adrenal gland may be done
• Filter/ Motion correction	: STD/Yes
• MPR/3D	: Coronal and sagittal/Nil
PHOTOGRAPHY	
• Window settings	: 350/50
• Printing format	: 17 × 14 –12 on 1 film for plain series
	: 17 × 1·4 –16 on 1 film for contrast series

SCT–PELVIS

INDICATIONS	: Ca cervix, bladder, rectum, prostate, Inflammation, trauma.
ENHANCEMENT TECHNIQUES	
• Oral	: 750 ml of 1.5-2% diluted contrast media may be given orally at a rate of 100 ml/10 minutes before the scan
• Rectal	: 500 ml

- Vaginal : Vagina may be packed with cotton/gauze soaked in diluted contrast media.
- IV-ml/ Delay : 100 ml-2 ml/sec- 60 sec delay.

PATIENT POSITIONING : Head first, supine

PATIENT INSTRUCTIONS : Absolute breath hold in mid-inspiration and to maintain the same level of breath on each instruction.

SCANOGRAM : Abdomen AP

REFERENCE LINE : Xiphisternum

SCAN REGION : Iliac crest to pubic symphysis.

SCAN PLANE : Axial

SCAN PARAMETERS

- Algorithm/ kV/mA : STD/120 kV/140 mA
- SFOV/Time : 35/2 sec
- Slice thickness : 10/10 pre-contrast from iliac crest to pubic symphysis. Post contrast 5/5

SPECIAL INSTRUCTIONS : Colonic preparation and air contrast is required for staging of rectal ca. Urinary bladder should be kept full during the scan (clamp the catheter if present). Delayed scan after contrast opacification of bladder may be require as the situation demands (bladder tumour, VVF, RVF etc).

IMAGE REVIEW : Additional scan for abdomen proper may be required depending on the findings

POST PROCESSING

- Recon algorithm/FOV : STD/35 cm depending on patient size. Targetted reconstruction with an FOV just to encompass the adrenal gland may be done
- Filter/Motion correction : STD/Yes
- MPR/3D : Coronal and sagittal/Nil

PHOTOGRAPHY

- Window settings : 350/50
- Printing format : 17 × 14 –12 on 1 film for plain series
  : 17 × 14 –16 on 1 film for contrast series

SCT–HIP

INDICATIONS : Trauma, osteonecrosis, tumour, infection, inflammation, trauma.

ENHANCEMENT TECHNIQUES
- Oral : Nil
- Rectal : Nil
- IV-ml/ Delay : Nil

PATIENT POSITIONING : Head first/Supine.

SCANOGRAM : Pelvis AP.

SCAN REGION : Iliac crest to pubic symphysis.

SCAN PLANE : Axial.

SCAN PARAMETERS
- Algorithm/kV/mA : STD/120 kV/140 mA
- SFOV/Time : 35/2 sec
- Slice thickness : 10/10 from iliac crest to roof of acetabulum. 3/3 from roof to inferior border of acetabulum. 10/10 from acetabular floor to ischial tuberosity

SPECIAL INSTRUCTIONS : If the patient is investigated for avascular necrosis 3/3 mm scan from roof to floor of acetabulum is good enough.

IMAGE REVIEW : Additional scan for abdomen proper may be required depending on the findings.

POST PROCESSING
- Recon algorithm/FOV : Bone/35 cm depending on patient size. Targetted reconstruction with an FOV just to encompass individual hip joints separately may be useful
- Filter/Motion correction : Sharp/Yes
- MPR/3D : Coronal and sagittal/If possible especially in trauma.

PHOTOGRAPHY
- Window settings : 2000/750
- Printing format : 17 × 14 –16 on 1 film for plain series

SCT–SI JOINTS

INDICATIONS : Sacroiliac arthritis

ENHANCEMENT TECHNIQUES
- Oral : Nil
- Rectal : Nil
- IV-ml/ Delay : Nil

PATIENT POSITIONING : Head first/supine with knee flexed slightly.

SCANOGRAM : AP pelvis. Table position adjusted so that sacrum is in the center.

SCAN REGION : S1 vertebrae to lower sacroilliac joint

SCAN PLANE : Axial with 20 degree forward angulation

SCAN PARAMETERS

- Algorithm/kV/mA : Bone/120 kV/140 mA
- SFOV/Time : 35/3 sec
- Slice thickness : 2/5 mm

IMAGE REVIEW :

POST PROCESSING

- Recon algorithm/FOV : Bone/20 depending on patient size.
- Filter/Motion correction : Sharp/Yes
- MPR/3D : Nil/Nil

PHOTOGRAPHY

- Window settings : 350/50
- Printing format : 17 × 14 –12 on 1 film for plain series
  : 17 × 14 –16 on 1 film for contrast series

SCT–LUMBAR SPINE

INDICATIONS : Degenerative disease

ENHANCEMENT TECHNIQUES

- Intrathecal : 5 ml iohexol 300 mg. Patient is asked to roll around on the table 3-4 times to mix the contrast well with CSF in thecal sac.

PATIENT POSITIONING : Head first/supine

SCANOGRAM : Abdomen lateral.

SCAN REGION : L1 to S1.

SCAN PLANE : Axial

SCAN PARAMETERS

- Algorithm/ kV/mA/Time : STD/120 kV/140 mA/3 sec
- SFOV/TIME : 35/3 sec
- Slice thickness : Two 5 mm sections along pedicle and sub-pedicular region of L1 to S1. Three 3 mm sections obtained through the center of the disc space and both end plates parallel to the end plate.

SPECIAL INSTRUCTIONS : Appropriate angulation to be given so that all sections are parallel to the end plates.

IMAGE REVIEW : Look for optimum contrast opacification of the thecal sac.

POST PROCESSING

- Recon algorithm/FOV : STD for disc. Bone for body sections/15 mm targetted reconstruction with an FOV just to encompass the vertebrae may be done
- Filter/Motion correction : Sharp/Yes
- MPR/3D : Nil/Nil

PHOTOGRAPHY

- Window settings : 350/50
- Printing format : 17 × 14 –12 on 1 film for plain series
  : 17 × 14 –16 on 1 film for contrast series

POST PROCESSING

- Recon algorithm FOV : STD for disc : Bone for vertebral body sections/targeted reconstruction with an FOV just to encompass the vertebra may be done
- Filter/Motion correction : Sharp/Yes
- Reformation/3D : Nil/Nil

PHOTOGRAPHY

- Window settings : 350/50
- Printing format : 17 × 14 –12 on 1 film for plain series
  : 17 × 14 –16 on 1 film for contrast series

SCT–SPINE

INDICATIONS : Trauma, tumour of the cord or spine, inflammation, paravertebral pathology.

ENHANCEMENT TECHNIQUES

- Intrathecal : 7-10 iohexol 300 mg. Patient is asked to roll around if possible on the table 3-4 times to mix the contrast well with CSF in thecal sac.

PATIENT POSITIONING : Head first, supine: neck flexed, shoulder depressed, buttocks raised.

SCANOGRAM : Lateral spine

REFERENCE LINE	:
SCAN REGION	: Region of interest. Include one vertebra above and below.
SCAN PLANE	: Axial
SCAN PARAMETERS	
• Algorithm/kV/mA/Time	: STD/140 kV/140 mA/3 sec
• SFOV/TIME	: 25/3 sec
• Slice thickness	: Contiguous 3-5 mm through the predetermined area.
SPECIAL INSTRUCTIONS	: Appropriate angulation to be given so that all sections are parallel to the end plates.
IMAGE REVIEW	: Look for optimum contrast opacification of the thecal sac.
POST PROCESSING	
• Recon mode FOV	: STD for disc/bone for vertebral body sections/targetted reconstruction with an FOV just to encompass the vertabra may be done
PHOTOGRAPHY	
• Window settings	: 350/50
• Printing format	: 17 × 14 –12 on 1 film for plain series
	: 17 × 14 –16 on 1 film for contrast series

CHAPTER 15

Three-Dimensional CT

1. DEFINITION

3D CT can be defined as the ability to visualize CT images in 3-dimensional profile.

2. INTRODUCTION

Spiral CT is a volumetric data acquisition study, which is well suited for 3D imaging of contrast opacified vascular structures, bones and soft tissues. Post-processing of CT scans refers to computer manipulations of scan data after slices are acquired and stored. These manipulations include MPR and 3D methods. MPR (multiplanar reconstruction) produces new slices from a set of CT scan sections. 3D methods produce realistic images that often look similar to photographs of anatomic specimens. MPR and 3D reconstructions are generated using special computer graphics software available on the scanner itself or on imaging workstation.

Contiguous axial or coronal images of the part in question are stacked together to produce a volume. In general, the collection of scans has been completed before 3D reconstruction is attempted. The entire set of slices must be available on a disk storage unit in the CT scanner or workstation. A command is given to read the CT scan slices and produce images according to a previously specified protocol or through operator interaction with a display console.

Stand-alone workstations consisting of a display unit, keyboard and interactive devices such as a stylus and pad, mouse or track ball are often available as accessories to CT scanners. Many 3D imaging workstations offer much higher performance and more interactive capability, which permit the user to specify and modify the types of images to be produced. Workstations have the advantage of greater flexibility and more functions, but often require extra training and add complexity to the task of generating 3D images.

3. PROCEDURE

To produce 3D images, the operator must select the orientation of the view (e.g. front, rear, top), threshold and lighting characteristics for the surfaces. Of these, the selection of threshold has the most pronounced effect on image quality. A low threshold setting (–150 HU) delineates the soft tissue surface and a higher one (+150 HU) isolates the bones. In advanced 3D reconstruction systems, it is possible to use transparency and show both the soft tissue and bony elements simultaneously.

The quality of 3D images depends on originally acquired scan data. So optimization of data is a pre-requisite for quality 3D rendering. If we have to perform 3D studies, we have to address in anticipation issues like relevant data acquisitions, contrast administration and reconstructions. In addition, we must have full knowledge of available rendering technique and tools for editing.

The 3D imaging in SCT calls for understanding of the following :

1. Spiral data acquisition
2. Contrast administration
3. Data processing
4. Confirmation of satisfactory data
5. Editing techniques
6. Selection of rendering techniques
7. Image display printing.

Spiral data acquisition

Spiral CT provides volumetric data which can be reconstructed at arbitrary intervals. Anatomic coverage and acquisition time dictate other acquisition parameters. Table travel distance depends on the anatomic coverage of the part under study, while acquisition time depends on the table speed. The shortest gantry rotation time available must be selected. Pitch selection (ideally between 1.0 and 2.0) depends on the effective section thickness and collimation. Helical CT permits volumetric scan and acquisition of continuous data is possible. It allows arbitrary reconstruction to generate overlapping images. FOV is selected as small as possible to minimize pixel size by excluding non-pertinent peripheral structures. Patient is instructed to have same level of inspirations during the study and he is coached to have adequate hold of breath. Better to keep 30 sec as upper limit because of difference to hold breath more than that.

Contrast administration

To ensure maximal vascular opacification, contrast medium bolus delivery duration must be equal to scan duration. Contrast medium volume (ml) = Contrast medium flow rate (ml/sec) × scan duration. For average patient weighing 60-80 kg, 3-4 ml/sec contrast medium delivery is ideally suited for optimal opacification of arterial system fit for 3D study. For angiography study (CTA), one more factor is to be considered (scan delay time) in order to ensure exact coincidence of SCT acquisition with contrast medium enhancement plateau in arteries of interest. To achieve this, the circulation time for contrast medium to travel from injection site to target anatomy is to be determined individually, generally 15-25 seconds. This scan delay time is suited for patients below age of 50 years and about 30-40 seconds in those who are above 50 years of age. An accurately timed contrast bolus is important for achieving maximal target vessel opacification while minimizing venous and parenchymal opacification throughout the duration of the spiral scan. To ensure consistent arterial opacification throughout the spiral acquisition, the bolus duration is made equivalent to the scan duration. Successful studies rely on preferential arterial enhancement and minimization of venous and parenchymal enhancement. Accurate timing is essential. Optimal delay time is determined by small test dose followed by dynamic images at 2 sec interval (non-incremental)—time-density curve may be generated to determine scan delay. Some manufactures provide bolus-tracking software such as smart prep (GE), which automatically triggers scanning once density increases in ROI. Non-ionic contrast media 300 mg/ml is preferred to avoid nausea and, vomiting. Bolus duration is equivalent to scan duration. Minimum of 2 cc/sec must be given. Scan of thorax may be done in caudocranial direction to avoid artifact from great veins or use higher volumes of low concentration contrast.

For the majority of abdominal and thoracic applications, the bolus duration is 30 sec. In performing thoracic CT angiography, an additional consideration is that the rapid inflow of iodinated contrast material can result in very high attenuation values (greater than 2000 Hounsfield units (HU)) with in the subclavian vein, bracheocephalic, or superior vena cava. Streak artifact resulting from this high intravascular iodine concentration can obscure subclavian arteries, the origin of the great vessels, or the ascending aorta. It may be advantageous in these situations to use higher volumes of lower concentration contrast to minimize this effect. An alternative solution may be to acquire the spiral CT scan in a caudal to cranial direction to allow the high concentration contrast to be cleared from the upper thoracic veins.

Reconstruction (data processing)

Continuity of the spiral CT data enables axial sections to be reconstructed at any point along the spiral path and at arbitrary intervals. It will result in smoother 3-D rendering, reduced partial volume artifact, and improved partial volume artifact. Although axial CT sections can be generated at arbitrary intervals, section thickness remains constant and is determined by the collimator width, scan pitch, and interpolation algorithm. The interpolation algorithm is a mathematical process that converts the spiral data into axial sections. In general, interpolation algorithm that requires a longer portion of the spiral path to generate an axial image will result in a wider section and a higher signal to noise ratio. Interpolation algorithms requiring less spiral data for image reconstruction will result in thinner, higher resolution sections but with a low signal to noise ratio. The aim is to produce images, which resemble conventional angiogram in which vessels are projected and viewed from an infinite number of directions. At first overlapping sections are obtained by reconstructing them at intervals usually half a collimator thickness. Highly attenuating structures like bone and metal can obscure target anatomy masking lower attenuation vessels. Manual or semi automated editing techniques can be used to remove higher attenuating structures prior to rendering MIPS. In manual technique ROI are drawn by the operator on an axial image to select the structures that should be included or excluded. Manual editing is time-consuming. Semiautomated techniques employ 3D connectivity based editing techniques to identify contiguous pixel within a threshold range. A seed is planted manually on a representative section with the region to be excluded. The seed is then allowed to grow into adjacent pixels within the prescribed threshold range. Once identified the pixels are assigned a 1000 HU value. The special attention required when reconstructing images for 3D purpose are :

- Reconstruction in soft algorithm
- Use smallest possible DFOV just to include the area under study
- Obtain overlapping images by reconstruction at smaller increment (at least 50% of collimation width)

Satisfactory data

3D imaging is sensitive to any patient motion during the scanning process, whether this occurs as the scans are acquired or not. If it is possible to obtain high-quality MPR images from a set of CT scan data in the coronal and sagittal orientations the same data set is usually acceptable for 3D imaging. The views that are most often generated by 3D imaging include frontal, lateral, top, bottom, rear, oblique and certain specialized views, according to the particular clinical needs of specific patients. The reconstruction is often much more successful at extracting bony surfaces and skin surfaces than at distinguishing among the muscle and facial layers of tissues because the difference between skin and air or between soft tissue and bone is high in CT scans. The differences among fat, muscle and other soft tissue types are relatively small, so they are more difficult to detect and display. This means that 3D display of CT scans is most often used for skin surface and bony surface display.

Optimising Editing Techniques

The efficiency of accurate 3D visualization is determined by striking a balance between the choices of using editing technique vs. non-editing techniques. Editing can vary from a quick, simple, interactive cut plane selection to a time consuming, meticulous 2D ROI selection, with intermediate 3D-ROI editing, region growing, and slab edit. A 3D ROI editing is done after a ROI is selected. This selected ROI is either removed or exclusively rendering. This requires the drawing of a single ROI, which can be applied to many cross-sections. The easiest way to perform this type of edit is to create a MIP from above and below that allows a cleavage plane to be identified between two structures. But this type of editing is insufficient to remove the pelvis/skull/large rib-cage parts, where line of cleavage cannot be identified. Highly attenuated structures such as bone, metallic implants, or intensely enhancing parenchyma, can mask target anatomy on MIPs and some SSDs. Because the MIP selects only the brightest pixel along each ray, a high attenuation structure anywhere along the path of the ray will dominate and thus mask a structure of lesser attenuation. Alternatively, surface rendering have the property of occlusivity. A less attenuating structure will be if its attenuation falls above the selected threshold. Before generating MIPs either manual or semiautomatic techniques must be used to remove the high attenuating structures. This technique can be time consuming, it allows greatest degree of control over what structures are included or excluded in the rendering. A faster approach to manual segmentation that removes some control is to divide the imaging volume into multiple slabs and perform a craniocaudal MIP on each slab. A region of interest is drawn on each slab and then extended into all individual axial sections represented in the slab. Semiautomated segmentation techniques use 3-D connectivity to identify contiguous pixels within a threshold range.

3. SELECTION OF RENDERING TECHNIQUES

Different rendering techniques are available. However all of them need not be applied in all cases. Selection of appropriate rendering method to address a particular problem is very essential.

Different rendering methods are described below :

I. **MPR :** The process that accomplishes the reformation of transaxial slices into coronal, sagittal or paraxial (any other arbitrary orientation) is called multiplanar reformation (MPR). It is a convenient method for displaying data. The limitation is that all visualized structures must lie in a single plane, which is practically impossible in 3D study to demonstrate a structure in its entirety, lest pseudostenosis are created. This problem can be solved by using the curved planar reformations (CPR), which are capable of demonstrating an un-interrupted longitudinal cross section, as the display plane curves along structure of interest. CPR are created from points that are manually positioned in any type of visualization, be it MPR, MIP, SSD, or VR. The CPRs are useful in displaying interiors of tubular structures such as bowels, etc, as well as structures immediately close to these lumens, such as mural thrombus/extrinsic neoplasia. In accurate, insufficient CPR points will result in a slipping off structures. Coronal sagittal or oblique single voxel thick planes are created from the stacked axial images. They display images along a single plane. Curved reformations are used to display bones, vessels and structures. These images retain all information concerning relative X-ray attenuation by tissues in the imaged volume. They are useful to show the wall of an aneurysm. Distances and relative positions of structures should not be assessed from these images.

II. **SSD (Surface Shaded Display) :** SSD provides perfect 3D representation of anatomy, relaying on gray scale to encode surface reflections from an imaginary source of illumination. The majority of clinical workstations (WS) display single surface renderings, with user selected thresholds. Some WS allow several thresholds to be defined and displayed with different coloured surfaces, as per encoding of different tissues. For each classification, data segmentation is required, both in threshold and editing, which in turn increases the processing time, but it is worthwhile. SSD images are generated after selection of an arbitrary user defined threshold. All voxels in individual slices above a particular threshold are selected to be included in 3D image and set white. Voxels with attenuation values less than the threshold are set black. It is an all or none phenomena. Usually only 10% of the available information on axial images is incorporated into the 3D image. So it is best for bone, skin, and contrast filled vessels. Contiguous pixels above the threshold are modeled as a single 3D structure by the computer. An imaginary source of illumination is thrown on the surface by the computer in order to depict surface reflections, which are encoded in image gray scale. This image can be set to rotate or tumble in space permitting one to view the image from any perspective. SSD's can be made with multiple threshold levels and colorized displays to enable segmentation of structure with varying attenuation. Since depth resolution between structures is preserved, overlapping vessels are well depicted. Majority of information regarding relative X-ray attenuation is lost in the threshold process. The limitation of the technique is that selection can affect the appearance of vascular stenosis dramatically and that structures within the threshold range with different attenuations like calcium, luminal contrast or metallic stents cannot be differentiated. Artificial colouring is possible in new machines.

III. **MIP (Maximum Intensity Projection) :** MIPs are generated by selecting a view angle along which x-rays are passed through the volumetric data set. The maximum value encountered by each ray is encoded in a 2D projectional display (brightest pixels in an imaginary plane are selected, illuminated and projected). MIP gray scale reflects relative x-ray attenuation. These projected images can be oriented in any anatomic plane including standard projections or in nonstandard orientations that rotate about a major anatomic axis. When rotated about an imaginary axis MIPs can be viewed in a cine loop fashion giving the appearance of continuous rotation of the object about this axis. No thresholding is done and hence the subtle variations in attenuation can be appreciated. This method is best used for angiography images to see vessels in three dimensions. MIP parameters can be varied to change the appearance of the image significantly. Vessel calcification affects evaluation of caliber and stenosis. A disadvantage of MIP is that depth resolution cannot be appreciated from a single projection. Multiple views can be generated in a cine loop to enable appreciation of depth relationships.

IV. **VR (Volume Rendering) :** It is the most complex among all rendering techniques. In this, all voxel values are assigned opacity levels that vary. Lighting effect can be simulated in a fashion similar to that with SSD, but there is no surface definition with VR, because lighting effects are applied in VR based on the spatial gradient. As lighting effects and variations in transparency are simultaneously displayed, it is better to view VR in colour by encoding different voxel values. Volume rendering uses the entire volumetric data obtained during spiral CT to produce a volume 3D image. Interactive thresholding allows visualization of different tissues and the differentiation between different tissues is based on this principle. The tissues incorporated based on the threshold are not on an all or non-basis. Thus allowing liver and portal vein together to be seen separately if the thresholds are adjusted accordingly. It is best used for bone, vessels and high contrast structures. Colouring is interactive and the shades of colour actually depict the kind of tissue being visualized. The opacity can be varied to see through superficial structures into the deeper layers. The gradients can be changed to change the contrast between differing tissues. Since the images are seen in real time video movies can be generated. It uses the entire volumetric data obtained during spiral acquisition to produce 3D image. It is best for bone, vessels and high contrast structures. It is not based on all or none basis. Endoluminal views are also possible by this rendering.

V. **Virtual Endoscopy :** Creation of virtual images has been possible for a long time but was restricted due to the non-availability of adequate computing power and cost of such computers. With the rapid advances in computers and image processing methods this has become possible on microcomputers. Creation of virtual endoscopic views is now possible on most of the computer systems supplied by the major medical imaging system vendors and even on PC systems bought from the market and software provided by the vendors who specialize only in image processing software. Rapid advances in imaging systems have made possible acquisition of large volume of data within a short interval of time to eliminate motion artifacts. In addition sections can be reconstructed within the desired degree of overlap. This significantly increases the resolution possible in the Z-axis, which is so essential to create virtual images with adequate resolution to be useful for diagnostic purposes.

Technical Considerations

It is possible to create virtual endoscopic views from any data, which consist of symmetric sections of the body. The other requirements are high contrast difference between the wall and lumen of the structure being depicted; this may be with air or contrast if CT is being used. Motion causing misregistration is eliminated by short acquisition times using fast spiral CT so as to complete the imaging within a single breath hold. Smooth muscle relaxants like Glucagon or Buscopan are used when bowel is being evaluated to stop peristaltic motion and to ensure adequate distension. Adequate XY-axis resolution is not a problem any more when using state of art CT equipment. The critical requirement is in the Z-axis, where generating overlapping sections minimizes partial volume averaging artifacts. When using spiral CT it has been found that the slice thickness is more critical than the spiral pitch in determining the Z-axis resolution. Segmented reconstruction of the CT slices gives a thinner slice profile than full reconstruction and the added image noise does not significantly affect the virtual rendering. Overlapping sections with 75% overlap are better than a 50% overlap.

Methods of virtual rendering

Surface shaded display defines the edges of the surface being viewed. The rays are cast from the viewing point within the lumen of the structure and are terminated where it intersects a voxel with attenuation higher than the threshold set by the operator. These voxels form the displayed surface and are displayed as white (or any colour). After all the voxels are defined, the image depth is shaded so that the surfaces further away from the viewing point appear darker. This technique is simple to use, quick and less memory intensive but displays only the surface and is more sensitive to noise. Volume rendering techniques define different attenuation structures within the volume. The rays are cast from the viewing point and the operator defines the degree of transparency of the structures of different attenuation that the rays meet, the images so created are more realistic, less sensitive to noise but are memory intensive and hence slow unless the computer has a large memory.

Applications

Virtual Colonoscopy

The indication is for screening for colonic cancer in patients with polyps, which necessitates repeated endoscopic surveillance. Good bowel preparation is essential because faecal matter can mimic polyps. Adequate colonic distention is also mandatory to avoid false positive diagnosis of cancer or strictures. Glucogon or Buscopan is given for bowel relaxation and air is used for distention of the colon. Scan parameters are 3-5 mm section thickness, 2 : 1 pitch to cover the region in single breath hold, segmented reconstruction at 1-1.5 mm interval to generate 200-250 images.

Virtual Bronchoscopy

The utility of virtual bronchoscope is in providing a road map for bronchoscopy and for planning transbronchial biopsy especially in regions where vessels are in close relation to the lesions. Stenosis and endoluminal masses can be elegantly displayed and in some situations can obviate endoscopy altogether. The airway distal to the stenosis can be visualized. It is especially useful in situations of extrinsic compressions where causative lesion is well seen on the source images. The standard protocol uses 2 mm sections with a pitch of 2:1 so as to acquire the data in a breath hold with segmented reconstruction at 1 mm intervals. An offshoot of the helical CT is the use of dynamic CT in assessment of tracheomalacia where the collapse of the trachea during expiration can be well appreciated.

Virtual Nasopharyngoscopy

The anatomy can be displayed on the endoscopic display, which is identical to the view of the surgeon during the surgical procedure. The myriad of variations of the osteomeatal complex can thus be anticipated pre-operatively

Virtual Angioscopy

An endoscopic view adds to the display of the abnormalities, especially in aneurysms and identification of vessel ostea. It also provides an elegant display of the stenosis and ulcerations in intimal plaques.

Merits

1. The most attractive merit of virtual endoscopy is its noninvasive nature and hence it is easy to repeat and reproduce. Patient is free to go after data acquisition.
2. The source images see beyond the mucosal surface.

Demerits

1. It is virtual and not real.
2. The most useful indicators of disease on invasive endoscopy in the form of hyperemia, erosions, friability and edema are not depicted.
3. Operator dependent. A minor change in the threshold value could show a severe stenosis to be apparently more moderate or vice versa.
4. Other technical problems like inadequate distension of a segment of colon could be misinterpreted as disease.
5. Time consuming process.

IV. USES

Three-dimensional imaging is now well established for the examination of bony surfaces and is useful for the surgical planning and evaluation. This is especially true for craniofacial abnormalities or plastic surgery and orthopaedics.

- Orthopaedic abnormalities/Trauma
- Angiography
- Craniostenosis/Craniofacial anomalies
- Virtual endoscopy
  - Colonoscopy
  - Bronchoscopy

In most cases, the information given by 3D CT is already there on axial images. But 3D pictures improve one's ability to appreciate this information. The classic example is fracture of pelvis and acetabulum. Though the fractures are well seen on the axial image and coronal and sagittal reconstruction, to truly appreciate the pattern of injury a 3D CT is needed.

V. DIFFICULTIES IN 3D IMAGING

There are significant difficulties with CT scanning for 3D reconstruction that may arise from artifacts in the scan slices or among the set of slices. These include the following:

1. Beam hardening artifacts caused by the non-uniform attenuation of x-rays in the planar section.
2. Patient motion during the scanning procedure.

3. Missing slices.
4. Metallic components, especially tooth fillings and prostheses.
5. Non uniform slice thickness, magnification factors, or gantry tilt.
6. CT scanner malfunction.

3D PROTOCOLS

3D CT FACE

INDICATIONS : Trauma
ENHANCEMENT TECHNIQUES
- Oral : Nil
- IV-ml/Delay : Nil

PATIENT POSITIONING : Head first/supine
PATIENT INSTRUCTIONS : Immobalisation of the part
SCANOGRAM : Skull lateral up to C3
REFERENCE LINE : Parallel to OM line
SCAN REGION : Supraorbital ridge to inferior border of the mandible
SCAN PLANE : Axial
SCAN PARAMETERS
- Algorithm/ kV/mA : STD/140 kV/200 mA
- SFOV : 25 cm
- Slice thickness : 3 mm
- Table feed : 5 mm

IMAGE REVIEW :
POST PROCESSING
- Recon mode/FOV : Soft/19 cm
- Filter : Nil
- Reformation/3D : Yes

PHOTOGRAPHY
- Window settings : Appropriate to highlight 3D image
- Printing format : Less number of images in 1 film

3D CT HIP

INDICATIONS : Trauma to define fracture and its extent
ENHANCEMENT TECHNIQUES
- Oral : Nil
- IV-ml/Delay : Nil (may be used for CTA if indicated or if pelvic vascular injury may be suspected

PATIENT POSITIONING : Head first/supine

SCANOGRAM : AP pelvis

SCAN REGION : 2 cm above the acetabular roof to 2 cm below the acetabular floor

SCAN PLANE : Axial

SCAN PARAMETERS

- Algorithm/kV/mA : STD/140 kV/200 mA
- SFOV : 42 cm
- Slice thickness : 3 mm
- Table feed : 6 mm

IMAGE REVIEW :

POST PROCESSING

- Recon mode/FOV : Soft (1.5 mm)/35 cm
- Filter : Nil
- Reformation/3D : Yes

PHOTOGRAPHY

- Window settings : Appropriate settings to highlight 3D images.
- Printing format : Less number of images in 1 film

3D CT PELVIS

INDICATIONS : Trauma to SI joints, sacrum, iliac wings complex, pelvic fractures involving acetabulam

ENHANCEMENT TECHNIQUES

- Oral : Nil
- IV-ml/Delay : Nil (CM used only pelvic vascular injury is suspected)

PATIENT POSITIONING : Head first/supine

SCANOGRAM : AP pelvis

SCAN REGION : Top of iliac crest to symphysis pubis

SCAN PLANE : Axial

SCAN PARAMETERS

- Algorithm/kV/mA : STD/140 kV/200 mA
- SFOV : 42 cm/40 sec
- Slice thickness : 3 mm
- Table feed : 5 mm

IMAGE REVIEW :

POST PROCESSING

- Recon mode/FOV : Soft (1.5 mm)/35 cm
- Filter : Nil
- Reformation/3D : Yes

PHOTOGRAPHY

- Window settings : Appropriate settings to highlight the 3D image
- Printing format : Less number of images in 1 film

3D CT SHOULDER

INDICATIONS : Trauma

ENHANCEMENT TECHNIQUES

- Oral : Nil
- IV-ml/ Delay : Nil (angiography is planned to study vascular injury)

PATIENT POSITIONING : Head first/supine

SCANOGRAM : AP scout of the shoulder

SCAN REGION : Just above the AC joint to lower scapular tip

SCAN PLANE : Axial

SCAN PARAMETERS

- Algorithm/kV/mA : STD/140 kV/200 mA
- SFOV : 35 cm/40 sec
- Slice thickness : 3 mm
- Table feed : 7 mm

IMAGE REVIEW :

POST PROCESSING

- Recon mode/FOV : Soft (1.5 mm)/25 cm
- Filter : Nil
- Reformation/3D : Yes

PHOTOGRAPHY

- Window settings : Appropriate settings to highlight the 3D image
- Printing format : Less number of images in 1 film

3D CT KNEE

INDICATIONS : Trauma

ENHANCEMENT TECHNIQUES

- Oral : Nil
- IV-ml/Delay : Nil

PATIENT POSITIONING : Feet first/supine

SCANOGRAM : AP knee

SCAN REGION : 3 cm above the fracture site of the bone to 3 cm below the fracture site

SCAN PLANE : Axial

SCAN PARAMETERS

- Algorithm/kV/mA : STD/140 kV/200 mA
- SFOV : 20 cm
- Slice thickness : 3 mm
- Table feed : 5 mm

IMAGE REVIEW :

POST PROCESSING

- Recon mode/FOV : Soft (1 mm)/16 cm
- Filter : Nil
- Reformation/3D : Yes

PHOTOGRAPHY

- Window settings : Appropriate settings to highlight 3D images
- Printing format : Less number of images in 1 film

3D CT ANKLE

INDICATIONS : Trauma

ENHANCEMENT TECHNIQUES

- Oral : Nil
- IV-ml/Delay : Nil

PATIENT POSITIONING : Feet first/supine

SCANOGRAM : AP ankle

SCAN REGION : To cover the ankle joint

SCAN PLANE : Axial

SCAN PARAMETERS

- Algorithm/kV/mA : STD/140 kV/200 mA
- SFOV : 20 cm
- Slice thickness : 3 mm
- Table feed : 5 mm

IMAGE REVIEW :
POST PROCESSING
- Recon mode/FOV : Soft (1.5)/15 cm
- Filter : Nil
- Reformation/3D : Yes

PHOTOGRAPHY
- Window settings : Appropriate settings to highlight 3D images
- Printing format : Less number of images in 1 film

3D CT SPINE

INDICATIONS : Trauma
ENHANCEMENT TECHNIQUES
- Oral : Nil
- IV-ml/Delay : Nil

PATIENT POSITIONING : Head first/supine
SCANOGRAM : Lateral view of scanned spine part include cervical, dorsal, lumbar, sacral spine as required
SCAN REGION : 2-3 cm above area studied and 2-3 cm below the area studied
SCAN PLANE : Axial
SCAN PARAMETERS
- Algorithm/kV/mA : STD/140 kV/200 mA
- SFOV/Time : 25 cm/40 sec
- Slice thickness : 3 mm
- Table feed : 5 mm

IMAGE REVIEW :
POST PROCESSING
- Recon mode/FOV : Soft (1.5 mm)/15 cm
- Filter : Nil
- Reformation/3D : Yes

PHOTOGRAPHY
- Window settings : Appropriate settings to highlight 3D images
- Printing format : Less number of images in 1 film

CT BRONCHOSCOPY

INDICATIONS : Tracheobronchial abnormalities, especially in tracheomalacia

ENHANCEMENT TECHNIQUES
- Oral : Nil
- IV-ml/Delay : Nil

PATIENT POSITIONING : Head first/supine
SCANOGRAM : Chest AP
REFERENCE LINE : Sternal notch
SCAN REGION : To completely cover the tracheobronchial tree
SCAN PLANE : Axial
SCAN PARAMETERS
- Algorithm/kV/mA : STD/140 kV/130 mA
- SFOV/Time : 35 cm/1 sec
- Slice thickness : 2 mm
- Table feed : 4 mm

POST PROCESSING
- Recon mode/FOV : Soft/30 cm
- Recon interval : 1 mm
- Filter : Nil
- Reformation/3D : Yes

PHOTOGRAPHY
- Window settings : Appropriate settings to highlight 3D images
- Printing format : Less number of images in 1 film

CT COLONOSCOPY

INDICATIONS : Colonic neoplasia, polyps, strictures
ENHANCEMENT TECHNIQUES
- Oral : Nil
- IV-ml/Delay : Nil

PATIENT POSITIONING : Head first/supine
PATIENT INSTRUCTIONS : Good bowel preparation, absolute restriction of respiratory movement
SCANOGRAM : AP abdomen
REFERENCE LINE : At the level of xiphisternum
SCAN REGION : Xiphisternum to pubis symphysis
SCAN PLANE : Axial

SCAN PARAMETERS
- Algorithm/kV/mA : STD/140 kV/130 mA
- SFOV/Time : 42 cm/2 sec
- Slice thickness : 3 mm
- Table feed : 5 mm

IMAGE REVIEW :

POST PROCESSING
- Recon mode/FOV : Soft/35 cm
- Recon interval : 1.5 mm
- Filter : Nil
- Reformation/3D : Yes

PHOTOGRAPHY
- Window settings : Appropriate settings to highlight 3D images
- Printing format : Less number of images in 1 film

SPECIAL NOTE : Endoluminal view requires special software

CT ANGIOGRAPHY

The procedure of CT angiography requires rapid volumetric acquisition by spiral CT coupled with accurately timed high flow peripheral IV contrast injection. The resultant images are processed with computed rendering techniques to generate 3D images of the vasculature. The basics and principles of 3D imaging described above are applicable to vascular 3D imaging.

1. Clinical applications of CTA

1. Supplementary to conventional angiography.
2. Confirmation of an aneurysm suspected on CT/MRI/MRA.
3. Follow up of aneurysms.
4. To rule out serious vascular diseases.
5. Useful in seriously ill patients where conventional angio fails.
6. Patient refused for conventional angiogram.
7. Screening high-risk patients.

2. Image analysis and evaluation of stenosis

1. Review of reconstructed axial images, observation of small diameter vessels and accurate measurement of diameter using calipers.
2. Review of multiplanar images, helps to display anatomic relationship in a plane.
3. 3D image analysis.

Three-dimensional images are often unnecessary for diagnostic purpose. But it provides beautiful multidirectional demonstration of vascular anatomy similar to angiography. Small vessels may be rėmoved inadvertently during reconstruction. All vessel diameters should be measured from axial images only but it may not help if a vessel is narrowed in a non-axial direction.

3. Angiography—comparative study

A. MR angiography

1. No contrast media.
2. Local signal voids can be created in regions of complex flow at branch points and stenosis. This may cause overgrading of stenosis.
3. Thorax and abdomen—respiratory movement and peristalsis can affect image quality.
4. Calcified plaque results in overestimation of stenosis.
5. Major advantage is that it does not require contrast media injection
6. Low contrast

B. CT angiography

1. Not susceptible to complex flow dynamics as it images luminal contrast only.
2. Location and morphology of calcium and metallic clips are demonstrated with respect to vessel lumen.
3. Less morbidity
4. Multiple viewing angles
5. Lower cost
6. Less invasive
7. Low contrast to noise ratio
8. Partial volume effects are great limitation
9. Overestimation of stenosis
10. Compared to conventional/DSA angiography CTA is a low-resolution angiogram
11. Limitation in length coverage due to difficulty in holding breath.

C. Conventional angiography

- High resolution
- Invasive
- More contrast media
- High cost
- More time consuming
- High contrast to noise ratio

4. Comparison between rendering methods

	Advantages	*Disadvantages*
MIP	1. Differentiate different density structures like calcification, thrombosis etc.	1. Vessel overlap may lead to confusion
	2. Accurate calculation of stenosis	2. Multiple views required
SSD	1. Display complex anatomic relationship in vessels overlap or tortuosity	1. Cannot differentiate structures above threshold range
	2. Could be visualized in different angles	2. Incorrect threshold results results in loss of significant vascular anatomy
MPR	Entire lumen, course thrombus and wall calcificatiion are well demonstrated	Inaccurate curve drawing imitate false impression of stenosis Distance should never be measured on MPR
VR	Image similar to catheter angiography, preservation of depth perception, X-ray attenuation of endoluminal views	Expensive computer is required

5. Pitfalls of CT angiography

1. Underestimation of stenosis—it can occur when the vessel is small and collimation is thick by overestimating the caliber of vessel.
2. Overestimation of stenosis.

ANGIOGRAPHY PROTOCOLS

CTA-CIRCLE OF WILLIS

INDICATIONS	: Aneurysms, dissections, AVM's, or arterial occlusive diseases
ENHANCEMENT TECHNIQUES	
• Oral	: Nil
• IV-ml/Delay/Rate	: 70-100 ml/25 s/3 cc/s
PATIENT POSITIONING	: Head first/supine
PATIENT INSTRUCTIONS	: Don't change the position of the head
SCANOGRAM	: Skull lateral up to C3
REFERENCE LINE	: Parallel to OM line
SCAN REGION	: Floor of sella to orbital ridge

SCAN PLANE	: Axial
SCAN PARAMETERS	
• Algorithm/kV/mA	: STD/140 kV/200-300 mA
• SFOV/Time	: 25 cm/40 sec
• Slice thickness	: 1 mm
• Table feed	: 1.5 mm
IMAGE REVIEW	:
POST PROCESSING	
• Recon mode/FOV	: Soft (.5 mm)/10-15 cm
• Filter	:
• Reformation/3D	: Yes. RIO or region growing can be used to remove anterior, posterior and lateral margins of the skull. If base of skull substraction is needed, then region growing can substract skull. However this can be difficult and may require additional localized RIO editing to disconnect skull base from vessels in some regions.
PHOTOGRAPHY	
• Window settings	: Appropriate window settings to highlight 3 D images
• Printing format	: Less number of images in 1 film

CTA-CAROTID ARTERIES

INDICATIONS	: Atherosclerotic occlusive disease/dissection
ENHANCEMENT TECHNIQUES	
• Oral	: Nil
• IV-ml/Delay/Rate	: 70-100 ml/25 sec/4 cc/s
PATIENT POSITIONING	: Head first/supine
SCANOGRAM	: Skull lateral up to C3
REFERENCE LINE	: Parallel to OM line
SCAN REGION	: C6-C3
SCAN PLANE	: Axial
SCAN PARAMETERS	
• Algorithm/kV/mA	: STD/140 kV/200-300 mA
• SFOV/Time	: 25 cm/20 sec
• Slice thickness	: 2 mm
• Table feed	: 5 mm

IMAGE REVIEW :

POST PROCESSING

- Recon mode/FOV : Soft (1 mm)/15 cm
- Filter : Nil
- Reformation/3D : Yes

PHOTOGRAPHY

- Window settings : Appropriate settings to highlight 3D images
- Printing format : Less number of images in 1 film

CTA–THORACIC AORTA

INDICATIONS : Aneurysm, dissection, mural haematoma/ ulceration, trauma, coarctation and other defects

ENHANCEMENT TECHNIQUES

- Oral : Nil
- IV-ml/Delay/Rate : 100-150 ml/15 sec/4 ml/s

PATIENT POSITIONING : Head first/supine

SCANOGRAM : AP chest/chest and abdomen

SCAN REGION : T1-L2

SCAN PLANE : Axial

SCAN PARAMETERS

- Algorithm/kV/mA : STD/140 kV/200-300 mA
- SFOV : 35 cm/40 sec
- Slice thickness : 3 mm
- Table feed : 5 mm

IMAGE REVIEW :

POST PROCESSING

- Recon mode/FOV : Soft (1.5 mm)/25 cm
- Filter : Nil
- Reformation/3D : Yes

PHOTOGRAPHY

- Window settings : Appropriate settings to highlight 3D image
- Printing format : Less number of images in 1film

CTA–PULMONARY ARTERY

INDICATIONS : Aneurysm

ENHANCEMENT TECHNIQUES
- Oral : Nil
- IV-ml/Delay/Rate : 100 ml/15 sec/3 ml/s

PATIENT POSITIONING : Head first/supine
SCANOGRAM : Chest AP/chest and abdomen
SCAN REGION : Aortic arch to 15 cm down to the arch
SCAN PLANE : Axial
SCAN PARAMETERS
- Algorithm/kV/mA : STD/140 kV/200-300 mA
- SFOV/Time : 35 cm/30 sec
- Slice thickness : 3 mm
- Table feed : 5 mm

IMAGE REVIEW :
POST PROCESSING
- Recon mode/FOV : Soft (1.5 mm)/25 cm
- Filter : Nil
- Reformation/3D : Yes

PHOTOGRAPHY
- Window settings : Appropriate settings to highlight 3D images
- Printing format : Less number of images in 1 film

CTA–ABDOMINAL AORTA

INDICATIONS : Aneurysm, atherosclerotic disease and dissection
ENHANCEMENT TECHNIQUES
- Oral : Nil
- IV-ml/ Delay/Rate : 100-150 ml/ 20 sec/ 3 cc/s

PATIENT POSITIONING : Head first/supine
SCANOGRAM : Abdomen AP
SCAN REGION : Lower T12 - Lower L4
SCAN PLANE : Axial
SCAN PARAMETERS
- Algorithm/kV/mA : STD/140 kV/200-300 mA
- SFOV : 35 cm/40 sec
- Slice thickness : 3 mm
- Table feed : 5 mm

IMAGE REVIEW	
POST PROCESSING	
• Recon mode/FOV	: Soft (1.5 mm)/25 cm
• Filter	: Nil
• Reformation/3D	: Yes
PHOTOGRAPHY	
• Window settings	: Appropriate settings to highlight 3D images
• Printing format	: Less number of images in 1 film

CTA-RENAL ARTERIES

INDICATIONS	: Renal artery stenosis/trauma/hematuria
ENHANCEMENT TECHNIQUES	
• Oral	: Nil
• IV-ml/Delay/Rate	: 100-150 ml/20 sec/4 cc/s
PATIENT POSITIONING	: Head first/supine
SCANOGRAM	: Abd AP
REFERENCE LINE	: Xiphisternum
SCAN REGION	: T11 to 15 CM down
SCAN PLANE	: Axial .
SCAN PARAMETERS	
• Algorithm/kV/ mA	: STD/140 kV/200-300 mA
• SFOV	: 35 cm
• Slice thickness	: 2 mm
• Table feed	: 3 mm
IMAGE REVIEW	:
POST PROCESSING	
• Recon mode/FOV	: Soft (1 mm)/15 cm
POSTPROCESSING	
• Recon mode/FOV	: Soft (1.5 mm)/25 cm
• Filter	: Nil
• Reformation/3D	: Yes
PHOTOGRAPHY	
• Window settings	: Appropriate settings to highlight 3D images
• Printing format	: Less number of images in 1 film

CTA-MESENTERIC ARTERY

INDICATIONS	: Mesenteric artery thrombosis/stenosis.

ENHANCEMENT TECHNIQUES

- Oral : Nil
- IV-ml/Delay/Rate : 100-150 ml/timed/4 cc/s

PATIENT POSITIONING : Head first/supine

SCANOGRAM : Abdomen AP

REFERENCE LINE : Xiphisternum

SCAN REGION : T12- L4

SCAN PLANE : Axial

SCAN PARAMETERS

- Algorithm/kV/mA : STD/140 kV/200-300 mA
- SFOV : 35 cm
- Slice thickness : 2 mm
- Table feed : 4 mm

IMAGE REVIEW :

POST PROCESSING

- Recon mode/FOV : Soft (1 mm)/25 cm
- Filter : Nil
- Reformation/3D : Yes

PHOTOGRAPHY

- Window settings : Appropriate settings to highlight 3D images
- Printing format : Less number of images in 1 film

CT ANGIOGRAM PROTOCOLS

	IV Contrast				From	To	Collimation	Table interval	Recon
	Rate	Amount	Delay	Duration					
Circle of Willis	3 ml/s	70-100 cc	25 sec	40 sec	Floor of sella	Orbital ridge	1 mm	1.5 mm/sec	0.5 mm
Carotid arteries	4 ml/s	70-100 cc	25 sec	20 sec	C6	C3	2 mm	5 mm/sec	1 mm
Thoracic aorta	4 ml/s	100-150 cc	15 sec	40 sec	T1	L2	3 mm	5 mm/sec	1.5 mm
Pulmonary arteries	3 ml/s	100-150 cc	15 sec	30 sec	Aortic arch	15 cm down	3 mm	5 mm/sec	1.5 mm
Abdominal aorta	3 ml/s	100-150 cc	20 sec	40 sec	Lower T12	Lower L4	3 mm	5 mm/sec	1.5 mm
Mesenteric arteries	5 ml/s	100-150 cc	timed	30 sec	T12	L4	3 mm	5 mm/sec	1.5 mm
Renal artery	4 ml/s	100-150 cc	20 sec	30 sec	Lower T11	15 cm down	2 mm	4 mm/sec	1 mm

CHAPTER 16

High Resolution CT

I. INTRODUCTION

High-resolution CT (HRCT) is a technique introduced in the mid-1980s as a result of significant improvements in the CT process and in computers. The technical aspects of HRCT have been described by a number of workers. There is no general agreement among investigators as to what constitutes a "high-resolution" CT study. A number of technical modifications are possible in obtaining an optimal study. The most important modifications of CT techniques, which make it "high-resolution" are:

- The use of thin collimation,
- Image reconstruction with a high-spatial frequency (sharp) algorithm,
- Increased kVp or mA technique,
- The use of a large matrix size, and
- Targeted image reconstruction.

However, not all of these are performed on a routine basis. Since most of the applications of HRCT are in connection with lungs, the following discussion on high resolution CT will be considering lung HRCT as the prototype. Only the essential points of other HRCT technique will be discussed as additional points.

II. TECHNIQUE

Scan collimation

Scanning with the thinnest possible collimation (1-1.5 mm) is essential if spatial resolution is to be optimized.

Reconstruction algorithm

With conventional body CT, scan data are usually reconstructed with a relatively low-spatial frequency algorithm, that smoothes the image, reduces visible image noise, and improves the contrast resolution to some degree. Reconstruction of the image using a high-resolution algorithm reduces image smoothing and increases spatial resolution, making structures appear sharper.

kVp, mA (mAs) and Scan Time

In HRCT, image noise is more apparent than with standard CT. High-resolution techniques, such as the use of a sharp reconstruction algorithm, in addition to increasing image sharpness, increases the visibility of noise in the CT image. Since much of this noise is quantum related and thus decreases with increased technique (number of photons), increasing the (kVp) or (mA) used during scanning, or increasing scan time can reduce noise and improve scan quality. Noise is inversely proportional to the number of photons absorbed, it is inversely proportional to the square root of the mAs. kVp and mA can be easily increased when obtaining HRCT, and this increase in technique can result in a reduction in visible image noise. Increasing scan technique also increases the patient's radiation dose.

Matrix size

The largest matrix available should be used routinely in image reconstruction, in order to reduce pixel size. The largest available matrix in our set up is 512 × 512 and usually not changable.

Field of view and the use of targeted reconstruction

Scanning should be performed using a field of view large enough to encompass the patients. Retrospectively targeting image reconstruction to a single lung instead of the entire thorax using a smaller field of view significantly reduces the image pixel size and thus increases spatial resolution. Image targeting is considered to be optional and is recommended only when optimal resolution is desired.

Image photography

Although the manner in which the images are photographed does not affect the actual spatial resolution of the image, proper photography is important in allowing the images to be interpreted accurately. The window level and width used for photography have a significant impact on the appearance of the lung parenchyma, and the dimensions of visualized structures. Subtle abnormalities are difficult to detect if the photographic technique used is not appropriate, and normal structures can be made to look abnormal.

III. SPATIAL RESOLUTION OF HRCT

There is a fundamental relationship between pixel size and the size of structure that can be resolved using CT. Current scanners are capable of providing scan data with spatial resolution of 0.5 mm. Structures smaller than the pixel size should be difficult to resolve theoretically. However this is sometimes possible. Interlobular septae as thin as 0.1 mm and arteries with a diameter of 0.3 mm are sometimes visible on HRCT using a small FOV. It is because of large difference in attenuation between soft tissue structures and alveoli and use of high spatial resolution algorithm. The ability of HRCT to resolve true lung structures depends on their orientation relative to the scan plane. Structures measuring 0.1-0.2 mm in thickness can be seen if they are largely oriented perpendicular to the scan plane and extend through the thickness of the scan plane or voxel. Similarly sized structures that are oriented horizontally within the scan plane will not be visible because of volume averaging with the air-filled lung that occupies most of the thickness of the voxel.

IV. CONTRAST RESOLUTION

Low-contrast resolution, or tissue resolution, is the ability of an imaging system to demonstrate small changes in tissue contrast. Contrast resolution can also be stated in terms of the ability of the CT unit to image very small objects that vary slightly in density from the environment in which they are located. Low-contrast resolution in CT is affected by several factors. These include photon flux, slice thickness, patient size, and sensitivity of the detector, reconstruction algorithm, image display, recording and noise. The photon flux depends on kVp, mAs and beam filtration. Whereas increasing the technical factors (kVp and mAs) increases photon flux, increasing the beam filtration and patient size reduces photon flux, because the radiation attenuation is greater. Another factor influencing low-contrast resolution in CT is slice thickness. In CT, collimation controls the slice thickness. Very thin slices require very narrow collimation. It is important to realize that as the slice thickness decreases the technical factors must be also increased. Detector sensitivity affects contrast resolution. CT detectors must be capable of discriminating among small differences in x-ray attenuation, which is required to measure small differences in soft tissue contrast. The low spatial frequency algorithm can be used for image smoothing which "may enhance the perceptibility of low-contrast lesions such as metastases". The size of the television screen and the viewing distance also affect contrast resolution. Finally, noise affects low-contrast resolution in CT. If too few photons are detected, then the image appears as "noise" and low-contrast resolution is degraded. To improve both contrast and spatial resolution, the dose must be increased so that more photons are available at the detector to generate stronger signals.

V. ARTIFACTS ON HRCT

Noise properties in CT

Noise in CT is the fluctuation of CT numbers from point to point in the image for a scan of uniform material, such as water. The noise level can be stated as a percentage of contrast or in CT numbers. The noise levels for CT scanners vary and depend on several factors including mAs, scan time, kVp, slice thickness, object size, and the algorithm. Noise in CT is mainly related to the following:

(1) Number of detected photons
(2) Matrix size (pixel size)
(3) Slice thickness
(4) Algorithm
(5) Electronic noise(detector electronics)
(6) Scattered radiation
(7) Object size.

If the width of the pixel size increases, the noise decreases, but spatial resolution also decreases. If slice thickness increases, noise decreases and spatial resolution decreases. If the dose increases, noise decreases.

Streak artifacts

Fine streak artifacts that radiate from the edges of sharply marginated high-contrast structures such as bronchial walls, ribs, or vertebral bodies are common on HRCT. On HRCT, streak artifacts are often visible as fine, linear, or dot-like opacities, that can be seen anywhere, but are most common overlying the posterior lung, paralleling the pleural surface and posterior chest wall. Streak artifacts can result from two separate mechanisms, "aliasing" and "correlated noise".

Motion artifacts

Pulsation or "star" artifacts are commonly visible, particularly at the left lung base, adjacent to the heart. With pulsation artifacts, thin streaks radiate from the edges of vessels or other visible structures, which therefore resemble stars, and small areas of apparent lucency may be seen between these streaks. These lucent areas, if not recognised as artifactual, may be mistaken for dilated bronchi. Also, the major fissure, usually on the left or other parenchymal structures such as vessels and bronchi, may be seen as double because of cardiac pulsation. This appearance can mimic bronchiectasis.

VI. RADIATION DOSE ASSOCIATED WITH HRCT

Since lung is the organ most frequently subjected to HRCT examination I limit the discussion on radiation dose to HRCT of lungs only. It has been made clear that HRCT as routinely performed results in a low-radiation dose as compared to conventional CT obtained with contiguous 1 cm collimation. In a more recent study using a scan technique of 120 kVp, 200 mA, 2 sec, the mean skin radiation dose was 4.4 mGy for 1.5 mm HRCT scans at 10 mm intervals, 2.1 mGy for scans at 20 mm intervals, and 36.3 mGy for conventional 10 mm scans at 10 mm intervals. Thus, HRCT scanning at 10 and 20 mm intervals, which is done in clinical imaging, results in 12% and 6%, respectively of the radiation dose associated with conventional CT. It has also been pointed out that obtaining low-dose HRCT (20 mA, 2 sec) at 20 mm intervals would result in an average skin dose comparable to that administered with chest radiography.

VII. HRCT OF LUNGS

Scan protocols

In obtaining clinical studies, the inspiratory level, patient position, and scan spacing can be varied. This may be determined by the clinical setting. Scans obtained with thicker collimation (5 mm) and expiratory scans may also be of value in certain situations.

Respiratory level

Routine HRCT is obtained during suspended full inspiration. Selected scans obtained following or during forced expiration may also be valuable in diagnosing patients with obstructive lung disease or airway abnormalities.

Patient position

Scans obtained with the patient supine are adequate in most instances. However, scans obtained with the patient prone are sometimes necessary for diagnosing subtle lung disease. Atelectasis is commonly seen in the dependent lung in both normal and abnormal subjects, resulting in so-called dependent density or subpleural line. These normal findings can closely mimic the appearance of early lung fibrosis, and they could be impossible to distinguish from true pathology on supine scans alone. However, if scans are obtained in both supine and prone positions, "dependent density" can be easily differentiated from true pathology. It has been further suggested that in patients with bronchiectasis angling the gantry 20 degrees caudally with the scan plane angled anteriorly and towards the feet improves visibility of the segmental and sub-segmental bronchi, by aligning them parallel to the plane of scan.

Scan spacing

Two fundamentally different approaches to HRCT have been used, at least partially determined by the indications for the scan. The first approach is to obtain HRCT at a few preselected levels, combined with a conventional CT study in which the entire thorax is imaged using contiguous 10 mm collimation scans. This technique is most appropriate when the primary indication for the study is an evaluation of the entire thorax. HRCT scans obtained at the levels of the aortic arch, carina, and at a level 2 cm above the right hemidiaphragm allow the assessment of the lung regions in which lung biopsies are most frequently performed.

The second approach is to obtain HRCT images only. There is no single correct HRCT protocol that should be used. Scans obtained at 1-cm intervals from the lung apices to bases to be the most appropriate routine scanning protocol, allowing a complete sampling of the lung and lung disease, regardless of its distribution. In patients who are likely to require prone images, scans can be obtained at 2-cm intervals from lung apices to bases, in both supine and prone positions. Since the prone and supine images will be slightly different, even if obtained at the same level, the number of images obtained will be equivalent to a supine position scan protocol using 1-cm spacing.

It may sometimes be appropriate to customize the number or location of scans, depending on the patient's suspected diseases, clinical findings, or the location of plain radiographic abnormalities. If the lung disease being studied predominates in a certain region of lung, as determined by chest radiographs, conventional CT, or other imaging studies, it makes sense that more scans should be obtained in the most abnormal area. In patients with suspected asbestosis, it has been recommended that more scans be performed near the diaphragm than in the upper lobes, because of the typical basal distribution of the disease, even if the chest radiograph does not suggest any abnormality in this region.

Photography

Level and width settings of approximately -700/1000 Hounsfield units (HU) would be appropriate for routine lung windows. Some authors prefer using an extended window width of 1500 to 2000 HU when viewing the lung, but this reduces contrast between lung parenchymal structures such as vessels and bronchi, and the air-containing alveoli. On the other hand, extended windows can be of value in detecting abnormalities of overall lung attenuation, and are also useful in evaluating the relationship of peripheral parenchymal abnormalities to the pleural surfaces. Images with a window mean of -600 to –700 HU and an extended window width of 1500 HU are appropriate for routine lung windows. A window of –500 to –700/2000 HU could also be employed, and is particularly useful when pleuro-parenchymal abnormalities are being evaluated. Low-window settings (–800 to –900) with narrow-window widths (500) can be valuable in contrasting emphysema or air-filled cystic lesions with normal lung parenchyma. Such a low-window mean, particularly combined with a narrow-window width, would make the lung interstitium appear much more prominent than it really is, and could make a normal case appear abnormal. This window would also result in an overestimation of bronchial wall thickness. Large images are much easier to read. A six on one format using 14 × 17 film is recommended for photography of lung window images in order to make the images large enough to view easily.

Low dose HRCT of lungs

The efficacy of "low-dose high-resolution CT" has been assessed in two recent studies using 120 kVp, 20 mA, 2 second and concluded that low dose HRCT yields anatomic information comparable to conventional HRCT in majority of patients without significant loss of spatial resolution. Since noise is usually a big problem in large patients (because more x-ray photons are absorbed by the patient) and in the posterior part of the image (because of photon absorption by the spine), it would be most important to use increased technical factors when studying large patients or patients with suspected posterior lung disease. Low dose HRCT technique should not be routinely employed for the initial evaluation of patients with lung disease, although it would be valuable in following patients with a known lung abnormality, or in screening large populations at risk for lung disease.

Use of expiratory CT

Recently, CT scans performed during or following expiration have been used to demonstrate air trapping in patients with diseases associated with airway abnormalities or findings of obstruction on pulmonary function tests. The use of expiratory CT has been reported in patients with emphysema, asthma, the Swyer James syndrome, the cystic lung diseases associated with histiocytosis X and tuberous sclerosis, and in patients with a variety of causes of large and small airway obstruction. In normal subjects, in most lung regions, lung parenchyma increases uniformly in attenuation during expiration, but in the presence of air trapping, lung parenchyma remains lucent on expiration and shows little change in volume. Differences in attenuation between normal lung regions and regions that show air trapping often measure more than 100 HU. In patients with obstructive lung disease, airways disease, or emphysema HRCT scans obtained during suspended respiration, following forced expiration, can show evidence of air trapping in the absence of morphologic abnormalities recognizable on inspiratory HRCT scans. Expiratory scans at three selected levels (aortic arch, hila, lower lobes) are generally sufficient for showing significant air trapping when present.

Use of spiral CT

The use of spiral or helical technique is not recommended for HRCT in patients with suspected diffuse lung disease. Obtaining scans with a spiral technique results in an increase in effective slice thickness, thus resulting in some loss of spatial resolution.

Dynamic ultrafast high-resolution CT

A technique termed Dynamic Ultra Fast High-Resolution CT (DUHRCT) has also been shown to be valuable in the diagnosis of air trapping. With DUHRCT, a series of fast HRCT scans are rapidly obtained as the patient forcefully exhales, in order to demonstrate dynamic abnormalities of lung attenuation and morphology that result from air trapping. DUHRCT studies have been performed using an ultrafast electron-beam CT scanner that is capable of obtaining HRCT images with a 100 msec scan time (3 mm collimation, 150 kVp, 650 mA).

VIII. TEMPORAL BONES

Introduction

The temporal bone pushes the limits of any imaging modality to its extreme because high-resolution images that have the ability to precisely characterize thin plates of bone, air, and a wide variety of soft tissues are required. Radiologists must be able to visualize structures with dimensions smaller than 1 mm such as the stapes or the endolymphatic sac. As important as visualizing osseous structures, temporal bone imaging also must be able to evaluate soft tissues such as blood vessels, venous sinuses, cerebrospinal fluid (CSF), and adjacent areas such as the parotid gland, nasopharynx and brain. The spectrum of pathology affecting the temporal bone is broad, and the symptoms are often quite nonspecific. Thus imaging must simultaneously be a good survey study and be a highly specific examination. Because these requirements must be met, several techniques may be required. Computed tomography (CT) is excellent for the evaluation of disorders that primarily affect the air spaces (cholesteatoma) or the cortical bone (otosclerosis). CT is also useful for evaluating the soft tissues in many lesions (paragangliomas). By comparison, magnetic resonance imaging (MRI) has limited ability to evaluate normal dense cortical bone and air because both give MRI signal voids. For this reason, unless there is pathology present, MRI cannot distinguish the air spaces from the thin bony septations of the middle ear and mastoid. However, if fluid fills the air spaces, MRI can provide limited information. MRI excels in the evaluation of the soft tissues, CSF, and blood vessels.

High Resolution CT

HRCT of temporal bone gives very good delineation of the structures of the middle ear, inner ear and internal acoustic canal. A few indications for its use are :

- To see the extent of erosion and ossicular integrity in case of cholesteatoma

- Case of sensorineural deafness to rule out otosclerosis
- In cases of trauma to look for ossicular integrity, involvement of inner ear and region of facial canal by the fracture line
- Suspected case of congenital anomalies
- Evaluation of vascular tinnitus etc.
- Also this procedure gives a road map, in case surgery is required in detecting the so called dangerous variants – naked (dehiscent) IJV, carotid artery which pouts into the middle ear cavity and presence of soft tissue in 'blind spots' to the ENT surgeon – Prussak's space and sinus tympani in case of cholesteatoma, which may be left behind in case its presence in these areas are not detected earlier which may lead to recurrence of cholesteatoma.

Technique

1-2 mm axial and coronal sections are studied as part of complete evaluation. This is essential because of the multidirectional orientation of the temporal bone structures. Axial images are obtained by tilting the gantry to be parallel to the line, which joins the superior orbital rim to the external auditory canal (30-degree upward angulation to the Reid's base line). This line is parallel to the lateral semicircular canal and displays the temporal bone structures to the best advantage. Compared with other planes this plane allows separation of the individual component of the temporal bone so that they are more completely seen with less overlap and fewer partial volume artifact. This position avoids radiation to the lens also. Coronal scans are obtained with the patient supine or prone with the neck completely extended. It is performed 120 degree above the anthropological base line.

IX. PARANASAL SINUSES (SCREENING SINUS CT)

Screening sinus CT is not a high resolution CT in the true sense. Even though 3 mm sections are taken they can be grouped under high resolution CT because 3 mm sections can provide adequate information concerned with osteomeatal complex and images are reconstructed in high resolution algorithm. Coronal CT is currently the modality of choice in the evaluation of the paranasal sinuses and adjacent structures. Its ability to optimally display bone, soft tissue and air facilitates accurate depiction of anatomy and extent of disease in and around paranasal sinuses. In contrast to standard radiographs, CT clearly depicts the fine bony anatomy of the osteomeatal channels. It is advised to perform the initial CT scan after a course of adequate medical therapy to eliminate reversible changes of mucosal inflammation and to better evaluate the underlying anatomic structures. Routine pretreatment with a sympathomimetic nasal spray15 minutes before scanning to reduce nasal congestion is recommended. This minimizes mucosal oedema and allows an improved display of the fine bony architecture and any irreversible mucosal disease.

Positioning

Because the coronal plane optimally displays the osteomeatal unit (OMU) and the relationship of the brain and ethmoid roof, as well as depicts the relationship of the orbits to the paranasal sinuses, imaging in the coronal plane is recommended. Because the coronal images closely correlate with the surgical approach, they should be obtained in all patients with inflammatory sinus disease who are endoscopic surgery candidates. Optimally the coronal study should be performed in the prone position, so that any remaining sinus secretions do not obscure the OMU. In patients who cannot tolerate prone positioning (children, patients of advanced age, etc.) the "hanging head" technique can sometimes be utilized. In this technique the patient is placed in the supine position, and the neck is maximally extended. A pillow placed under the patient's shoulders helps positioning. The CT gantry is angled as perpendicular as possible to the bony plate. It is not always possible to obtain direct coronal images with this technique.

Examination Protocol

The patient is placed prone, with the chin hyper-extended, on the bed of the CT scanner. The scanner gantry is angled as perpendicular as possible to the hard palate. The angulation of the scan plane is very important. Variations in scan angulation greater than 10^0 from the plane perpendicular to the hard palate result in significant loss of anatomic detail of the structures of the OMU. Scanning is performed as contiguous 3-mm thick images from the anterior wall of the frontal sinus through the posterior wall of the sphenoid sinus. Contiguous scans are obtained to avoid loss of information through "skipped" areas. The field of view should be adjusted to include only the areas of interest. This helps to reduce artifact from the teeth and associated metallic sructures and magnifies the small anatomic structures of the nasal cavity and adjacent paranasal sinuses. It is recommended to keep the exposure settings of 120 kVp and 160 mAs as optimal without compromising the image quality.

Image display

Windows are chosen to highlight the air passage, the bony detail, and the soft tissues. Usually a window width of +2000 Hounsfield units (HU) with a level of –200 HU are good starting parameters. The window width and level settings can then be manually manipulated to optimally display the anatomic detail of the uncinate process and ethmoid bulla, and once this is accomplished, these settings can be used to film the entire study.

X. BASE OF SKULL

HRCT of the skull base can be done to evaluate basal foramina's skull base erosions, fractures and CSF rhinorroea.

XI. OTHERS

HRCT can be done in any bony structures whenever fine details are essential for interpretation and diagnosis.

CHAPTER

17

Dual Phase CT of Liver

1. INTRODUCTION

In conventional contrast CT, liver is usually imaged in the venous phase or equilibrium phase. With the advent of fast spiral machines it is now possible to image the liver in the arterial and venous phase of contrast enhancement. This is called as dual phase biphasic/double pass spiral study. This noval idea made better detection and characterization of hepatic tumours possible.

2. BASIC PRINCIPLES

Liver has dual blood supply. 80% of its supply is provided by the portal vein and only 20% is from the hepatic artery. Most of the hepatic neoplasms derive their blood supply mainly from the hepatic artery. These neoplasms are therefore visualized more conspicuously as enhancing lesions in the arterial phase of hepatic enhancement prior to the circulation of contrast through the portal venous system. Detection of focal liver lesion depends on the attenuation difference between the lesion and normal liver parenchyma. A minimum attenuation difference of 10 HU is necessary for tumour detection.

The earliest intravenous contrast delivered to the liver is by the hepatic artery. This phase of contrast enhancement of the liver is called the hepatic arterial phase. It begins 20 seconds after the start of peripheral IV contrast injection. Since the hepatic artery contributes only 20-30% of the blood flow to the liver the enhancement of the normal liver parenchyma is minimal during this phase. Liver tumours which mainly receive their blood supply from the hepatic artery are seen as hyper-attenuating masses against the background of the normal minimally enhanced liver parenchyma in the hepatic arterial phase.

After the blood and IV contrast circulates the gut, it is delivered via the portal vein to the liver. This phase of contrast enhancement is called the portal venous phase. Since the portal veins contribute the remaining 70-80% of the hepatic blood flow the attenuation of normal liver parenchyma rises rapidly during this phase. Liver tumours which are not predominantly supplied by the hepatic artery and are hypovascular and best visualized in the venous phase as hypo-attenuating lesions against the background of the well enhanced normal liver parenchyma. The most common hypovascular tumours are metastatic lesions to the liver from primary adenocarcinoma of stomach, colon and pancreas. After the portal venous phase contrast from the interstitial spaces of liver parenchyma diffuses into the liver tumour. This combination of declining attenuation of normal liver parenchyma and increasing tumour attenuation results in the tumour becoming iso-attenuating to normal liver parenchyma and hence not detectable. This phase is called the equilibrium phase or delayed phase and occurs 90-120 seconds after IV contrast injection. Most often we image the liver in conventional contrast CT and dynamic CT in this equilibrium phase or in the venous phase when a lesion can be iso-attenuating and not detectable.

3. INDICATIONS

The common indications for dual phase CT of liver are :

1. Suspected hepatocellular carcinoma.
2. Hypervascular liver metastasis.
3. Detection of benign hypervascular lesions.
4. To characterize benign hypervascular lesions from malignant hypervascular lesions.

4. TECHNIQUE OF DUAL PHASE CT OF LIVER

After administration of oral contrast a plain study of the upper abdomen is done with collimation of 10 mm. This is followed by dual phase CT of the liver in the hepatic arterial and portal venous phase. 100 ml of 300 mg non-ionic contrast is administered with a pressure injector. An 18-gauge venflon is placed in the antecubital vein. The contrast is delivered at a rate of 3-4 ml/sec. The hepatic arterial phase of the study is acquired after a time delay of 20 secs from the onset of IV contrast injection. This is followed by the portal venous phase acquired after a time delay of 50-60 secs from the onset of IV contrast injection. The entire liver is imaged in both phases with a collimation of 5 mm and table feed of 7 mm followed by 3.5 mm retrospective reconstruction. For smaller lesions and for 3D reconstruction of the liver and hepatic vasculature thinner reconstruction intervals of 2 mm can be done. For certain lesions such as haemangiomas the liver can be scanned in the equilibrium or delayed phase also at 90 secs after the onset of IV contrast injection (triple phase study).

5. CLINICAL APLICATIONS

1. Hypervascular hepatocellular carcinoma and hypervascular metastasis isodense on venous phase are detected better in the arterial phase. They are seen as enhancing lesions against the normal liver parenchyma that has not yet enhanced with contrast.
2. The number of neoplastic nodules detected are more when the liver is imaged in both arterial and venous phases.
3. Pattern of enhancement of hepatic lesions in the arterial and venous phase is helpful in characterizing these lesions.

6. PITFALLS

In the hepatic arterial phase Transient Hepatic Attenuation Differences (THAD) are seen as lobar or segmental hypervascular areas due to extrinsic compression of portal vein by a tumour or occlusion of a segmental portal vein by a tumour thrombus. This leads to increased compensatory flow from the hepatic artery to that segment. THAD are typically wedge-shaped with straight margins and are peripherally located. They disappear in venous phase. A relative contraindication for dual phase CT of liver is poor cardiac output. It is difficult to determine the time delay for arterial and venous phase in these patients.

7. CONCLUSION

The sensitivity and specificity of dual phase CT in the detection and characterization of hepatic tomour is higher than conventional contrast CT or dynamic CT. Dual phase spiral CT should be the protocol of choice in CT evaluation of hepatic tomours.

CHAPTER

18

Dental CT

1. INTRODUCTION

Dental CT refers to a special software programme which allows us to evaluate the teeth and jaws. This software is constructed such that the multiple contiguous axial sections are fed into it to yield panoramic and para axial reconstructions. Paraxial reconstructions are reconstructions perpendicular to the planes of the tooth and are the only image which shows all cortices of the mandible well.

To perform implant procedure the oral surgeons and dentist need to know the precise height, width and contour of the alveolar process as well as its relationship to the maxillary sinus and mandibular canal. Before the development of CT dental reformatting programmes, attempts were made to obtain this information with panoramic, intraoral and cephalometric films. However panoramic film (OPG) produced up to 25% distortion making accurate measurements almost impossible. The width and thickness of the alveolar process cannot be determined in panoramic view. These drawbacks led to the need and development of dental CT.

2. TECHNICAL DETAILS

Axial images

Axial images are obtained with low kV and mAs settings (90-110 kV/120-160 mAs). Lateral scout is taken in supine position. 1 mm contiguous sections are obtained using bone algorithm. The mandible and maxilla have to be scanned separately. Mouth is kept open by placing a bite block in the mouth. The mandible is scanned parallel to the inferior cortex of the mandible. Maxillary images are obtained parallel to the hard palate. Gantry should not be angulated and hence a separate study is done for mandible and maxilla, as their angles are slightly different. All measures have to be taken to avoid movement including swallowing. An axial image is selected at the level of root of teeth demonstrating the full contour of the mandible or maxilla. A curved line is superimposed on the axial image by computer manipulation. This line defines the plane and location of the reformatted panoramic images.

Reconstruction

Reconstructions are obtained in both panoramic and cross-sectional views. The width of the cross-sectional images should be enough to show all the four cortices. A spacing of 2 mm is usually used between the reconstructed images. The reconstructions should cover all teeth from right third molar to left third molar. The reformatted cross-sectional images are defined by multiple numbered lines that the programme automatically deposits perpendicular to the curved line. Streak artifacts which degrade visualization of bone on direct coronal images do not degrade the reformatted cross-sectional images because the artifact is projected at the level of the crowns of the teeth and not over the bony alveolus. At the end of the programme three types of images are displayed.

1. Axial
2. Cross-sectional
3. Panoramic

Typically there will be approximately 30-50 axial images, 40-100 cross-sectional images and 5 panoramic images.

Filming

Life-sized cross-sectional and panoramic images are preferred. This can usually be accomplished using four 14 × 17 films. Most often the axial images are filmed with 12 images per sheet of film and the cross-sectional and panoramic images actually contain multiple images. The images can be photographed at a window width of 3000-4000 and a level of between 300-500. A millimeter scale displayed on the films is used to verify the degree of magnification and to obtain accurate measurements.

3. INTERPRETATION OF DENTAL IMAGES

Each CT view can be related to the other by a series of scale marks that appear on the film. Marks, which run along the side of cross-sectional and panoramic images, correspond to the direct axial slices that are used to reformat the images. OPG is extremely unreliable where measurements of the posterior maxilla are concerned. Life-size images allow accurate measurement to be made by the implantologist wherever he wants. The radiologist must markout the site of the mental foramen on both sides and indicate line mark wherever possible. The height and width of the alveolar process are measured for mandible and maxilla in different manner. In the mandible the height in the region distal to the mental foramen is measured from the top of alveolar process to the top of the mandibular canal. Measurements are provided from the top of alveolar ridge to the bottom of·mandible. In the maxilla the height in the distal aspect is measured from the top of alveolar process to the floor of the maxillary sinus. More anteriorly the height is usually not limited by the maxillary sinuses and is measured from the alveolar ridge to the nasal fossa floor.

The measurement from the top of the alveolar ridge to the top of mandibular canal is important so is the identification of the mandibular canal. The mandibular canal is very well visualized as a rounded "hole" on the cross-sectional images. For identification several methods are practised if it is not seen on cross sectional images. The cross-sectional image of the mandible demonstrates an indentation on the lingual cortex of the mandible called the cortical **niche sign** which is created by the mandibular nerve as it traverses the mandible. This sign is helpful in identifying the location of mandibular canal.

The triangulation method utilizes the scale marks on the films to relate an anatomic structure well seen on one view with location on another view i.e. the information from the panoramic and axial views can be utilized to identify the canal on cross sectional images. The right and left hemi-mandibles are symmetrical and the distance from the bottom of the mandible to the bottom of the canal on the right side at a particular point is the same as the distance measured at same point on the left. This information can be used to estimate the position of the canal on the opposite side if the other side is identified.

4. INDICATIONS

1) Pre-implant evaluation
2) Focal lesions
3) Miscellaneous
   a) Impacted teeth
   b) Supernumerary teeth

Pre-implant evaluation

Dental implants are metal posts that are surgically implanted in the jaw to support a fixed dental prosthesis in partially, or completely edentulous individuals. Each implant has a screw at the crown end on which 2-3 artificial teeth can be supported. The success of implant depends on the size of the implant, the available space and the condition of the underlying bone. The larger the implant the better is the eventual prognosis of the patient. To decide what size and width of the implant is to be used it is necessary to measure the height and width of the bone, where the implant is to be placed. Currently this is done by OPG, which only allows measurement of height and not of width. Moreover this measurement can be erroneous.

In totally edentulous patients, where all line marks are lost, special ball bearing or barium paste markers are used to help the implantologist localize the areas required on the patients. In partially edentulous patients, the remaining teeth aid in the process. Apart from these measures, the panoramic and paraxial images also correlate with each other, thus allowing us to place the Paraxial images in relation to the panoramic appearance of the teeth and OPG's if available.

Various types of alveolar edge configuration have been described in totally edentulous patients with significant bone loss and these are self-explanatory—rounded pointed, knife–edge. Usually as a rough rule, a height of 10 mm and a width of 4 mm is the minimum required for the smallest possible implant. Apart from these measurements, the images allow a qualitative assessment of the bone texture. If there is significant osteopenia, the implant may not hold leading to failure. Focal lesion such as cyst, periodontal erosive lesion and abscesses may further adversely affect the implant.

Focal lesion

Dental CT also allows us to evaluate focal lesions in the jaw. These include

a) Cyst such as dental or dentigerous cyst and odentogenic keratocysts
b) Neoplasms, such as ameloblastomas, odentogenic fibromas, fibrous displasias etc.
c) Other lesions such as buccal carcinoma, infections etc.

The role of dental CT in these situations allows us to assess the extent of involvement of the jaws and associated structures. Thus the following relationships are evaluated. (1) The relationship of the mandibular canal with the lesion. If the lesion is below the canal it is always non-odentogenic in etiology. (2) The extent of involvement of the lingual, buccal and alveolar cortices. In these situations, dental CT is not to be used on its own, but is a useful adjunct to contrast enhanced CT with 3D CT and routine reconstruction. In this situation thicker sections may be obtained for the panoramic and Paraxial reconstructions, unless the information requested is extremely critical.

Miscellaneous

In patients with impacted teeth of extreme molared, if the relationship of the teeth to the mandibular canal is suspected, a dental CT helps in evaluating the relationship quantitatively and in detail. Similarly prior to the extraction of supernumerary teeth on the placed impacted teeth, the use of dental Ct would allow to evaluate the relationship with various adjacents structures.

CHAPTER 19

Osteo CT (QCT)

I. SCANNERS

Quantitative CT (QCT) was introduced in 1980. The major step in overcoming imperfection of real CT scanner has been the introduction of calibration. 3rd generation CT scanners have a relatively well collimated detector aperture. Hence they are less susceptible to quantification and calibration errors caused by scatter artifacts compared to 4th generation.

II. TECHNIQUE

To determine bone mineral density the CT number of the patient is compared with a reference standard of known composition and density distribution. Calibration may be simultaneous or non-simultaneous. For simultaneous calibration patient is placed on top of a calibration phantom that has inserts of known mineral density running perpendicular to the plane of CT slices. In non-simultaneous calibration technique a quasianthropometric tissue equivalent calibration phantom is scanned before or after the patient. Four constituents of bone contribute significantly to x-ray attenuation, namely - bone mineral, organic bone matrix, haemopoetic bone marrow, and fatty bone marrow. In the presence of yellow marrow whose absorption properties are different from those of water, single energy QCT technique underestimates the actual bone mineral content. Dual energy technique allows for accurate determination of mineral content regardless of the amount of fat present and it allows accurate determination of fat content regardless of the BM content.

III. QCT OF THE SPINE

Vertebral density is measured by assessing representative volume of 2-3 ml of purely trabecular bone. The ability to measure that area selectively is advantageous because the turnover rate of trabecular bone is approximately 8 times that of cortical bone of spine. The patient is positioned at top of the calibration phantom. To avoid artifacts a bolus bag is used to fill the air gap between patient and phantom. Using a lateral scout view 10 mm scans are taken through midbody parallel to endplates of 3-4 vertebrae (T12-L4). For single energy QCT measurements a low dose low energy setting should be chosen. For dual energy QCT the lower energy setting should be as low as possible with an effective energy of about 40 kev. The upper energy should be as high as possible typically 120-140 kvp.

IV. CLINICAL APPLICATION

QCT has been used to model patterns of vertebral base diminution with ageing to estimate skeletal status in health and disease, to protect subsequent fracture risk and to monitor interventions. Estrogen replacement therapy initiated soon after the correction of ovarian function is universally accepted as an effective means of retarding bone loss and preventing fracture of spine and hip. QCT has been of great value in chronicling this period of rapid bone loss and substantiating the response to estrogen therapy. The estrogen dose of 0.6 mg/day is the lowest effective dose in abbreviating this rapid involution.

V. INDICATIONS FOR QUANTITATIVE CT

1. Assessment of patients with metabolic diseases known to affect skeleton.
2. Assessment of premenopausal women for initiating estrogen therapy.
3. Establishing a diagnosis of osteoporosis or assessing its severity in context of clinical case.
4. Serial assessment for monitoring down prognosis or therapeutic response.

Men are known to have more angular BMD than women but from around the 4th decade there is a gradual reduction in BMD in both sexes. In women this rate of loss accelerates at the time of the menopause and continues for 10-15 years. After this period the rate of loss is similar to that of men. It is known that one in four women and one in ten men will have at least one osteoporotic fracture by the age of 70 years. Clinical risk factor are assessed and bone densitometry performed if a number of risk factors are present.

CHAPTER

20

Multi-Slice CT (MSCT)

I. HISTORY

Since its clinical introduction in 1990, volumetric CT scanning using spiral scanners has resulted in a revolution for diagnostic imaging. In addition to new applications for CT, such as CT angiography and the assessment of patients with renal colic, many routine applications such as the detection of lung and liver lesions have substantially improved. Helical CT has improved over the past eight years with faster gantry rotation, more powerful X-ray tubes, and improved interpolation algorithms. However, in practice, the spiral data sets from monoslice systems suffered from a considerable mismatch between the transverse (in plane) and the longitudinal (axial) spatial resolution. Similarly, in routine practice, a number of limitations still remained which prevented the scanning protocol to be fully adapted to the diagnostic needs.

In 1994 introduction of sub-second scanner was a first step to facilitate routine clinical work with respect to scannable volumes, total scan time and axial resolution. Compared to that time standard 1 sec scanners, the 750 millisecond rotation time allows to scan 33% longer volumes or to correspondingly reduce the total scan time or to correspondingly improve axial resolution. The greatest advance has been the recent introduction of multislice CT (MSCT) scanners. In 1998, this new technology has been introduced by several manufactures representing an obvious quantum leap in clinical performance.

II. INTRODUCTION TO MSCT

Multislice CT can be seen as a continuation of the exciting innovation that was introduced by spiral CT. It is a technologic advancement that allows simultaneous acquisition of multiple images during a single rotation of the x-ray tube. One important advantage of multislice CT is the ability to rapidly scan large volumes while maintaining high Z-axis resolution. Many terms for this new CT techniques are used: "Multi-detector helical or spiral CT", "Multi-row detector helical/spiral CT". So far there is no generally accepted term for the modality.

Fundamental advantages of MSCT include :

- Substantially shorter acquisition time.
- Retrospective creation of thinner or thicker sections from the same raw data.
- Improved 3-dimensional rendering with diminished helical artifacts.

For example, a scanner with a 500 msec rotation time and the simultaneous acquisition of four slices offers an 8-fold increase of performance compared to previous 1 sec, single slice scanning. The key issue is correspondingly improved temporal resolution. In general terms, the capabilities of spiral CT can be expanded in various ways:

- To scan anatomical volumes with standard techniques at significantly reduced scan time; or
- To scan larger volumes previously not accessible in practical scan time; or
- To scan anatomical volumes with high axial resolution (narrow collimation) to closely approach the isotropic voxel of high-quality data sets for excellent 3-dimensional post processing and diagnosis.

III. HARDWARE CONSIDERATIONS FOR MSCT

Multiple detector arrays are a set of several linear detector arrays, tightly abutted. The multiple detector array is an assembly of multiple solid-state detector array modules. With a traditional single detector array CT system, the detectors are quite wide and the adjustable collimator determines slice thickness. With these systems, small motors under computer control adjust the spacing between the collimator blades.

With multiple detector arrays, the detectors determine slice width, not by the collimator (a collimator does limit the beam to the total slice thickness). To allow the slice width to be adjustable, the detector width must be adjustable. It is not feasible, however, to physically change the width of detector arrays per se. Therefore, with multislice systems, the slice width is determined by grouping one or more detector units together.

Multiple detector array CT scanners make use of solid-state detectors. For a third-generation multiple detector array with 16 detectors in the slice thickness dimension and 750 detectors along each assay, 12,00 individual detector elements are used. The fan angle commonly used in third-generation CT scanners is about 60°; so fourth-generation scanners require roughly six times as many detectors as third-generation systems. Consequently, all currently planned multiple detector array scanners make use of third-generation geometry.

It is easy to design a multi-slice scanner for a fixed slice collimation; the challenge is to design the detector in such a way as to meet the clinical requirement of different slice collimations adjustable to the diagnostic needs. There are basically two different approaches :

- The matrix detector with elements of a fixed size
- The adaptive array principle.

An example of a **matrix detector** is a detector divided into 16 small elements each providing a 1.25 mm thick slices at the centre of rotation. The outer detector rows cannot be used individually. The only way out is to sum the signals of the outer rows to generate thick slices. The detector dimensions are references to the scanner's isocentre, the point at the centre of gantry rotation. The electronics are available for four detector array channels, and one, two, three or four detectors on the detector module can be combined to achieve slices of 4 × 1.25 mm, 4 × 3.75 mm, or 4 × 5.00 mm. To combine the signal from several detectors, the detectors are essentially wired together using computer-controlled switches.

In summary, the matrix detector is well suited to scan at 4 × 1.25 mm collimation but not more than 4. Wider collimations 4 × 2.5 mm etc. can be realized by signal combination during read out but at the expense of dead zones and a corresponding waste of dose. The unnecessary mechanical cuts and optical separations between the small elements correspondingly reduce the geometrical efficiency and therefore, the dose efficiency of the system.

These arguments lead to the development of **Adaptive Array Detector (AAD)**. The design of the Adaptive Array Detector tales into account the cone beam constraints for optimal image quality, optimizes the dose efficiency and in conjunction with an Adapted Axial Interpolator (AAI) provides a flexible selection of slice widths. Narrow detector elements are closed to the centre; the width of the detector rows increases with distance from the centre. Unnecessary dead spaces are avoided and with the corresponding prepatient collimator and the proper read-out schemes the following combination can be achieved : 2 × .5 mm, 4 × 1 mm, 4 × 2.5 mm, 4 × 5 mm, 2 × 8 mm and 2 × 10 mm. These combinations represent the collimation of the X-ray beam at centre, e.g. (a) 4 × 5 mm collimation means an X-ray beam width at centre of 20 mm. Consequently with sequential imaging four 5 mm slices would be generated during one rotation.

In spiral imaging the variety of axial sampling patterns as a function of pitch allows both to obtain slice widths independent of pitch and to reconstruct a multiplicity of slice widths from a scan with collimation narrower than slice. To achieve this AAI-scheme provides a set of linear and nonlinear interpolars, which are adapted to the desired pitch, collimation and slice width. To give some examples from a spiral scan with 4 × 1 mm collimation slice widths of 1, 1.25, 1.5, 2, 2.5, 3, 4, 5 upto 10 mm can be obtained by adjusting the width and functional form of the interpolar. On the other hand, a selected slice width S, like S = 5 mm, may be obtained from different collimator settings, like 4 × 1 mm or 4 × 2.5 mm.

This is important to remember for clinical application, as the narrower collimation is preferable from image quality reason, i.e. the reduction of partial effects. Yet another design criterion should be emphasized, spiral scanning at large pitch, e.g. large table velocity, implies a more severe inconsistency between direct projections, taken half a rotation later with a quarter offset. The reason is changing anatomy in axial direction, which is particularly pronounced for large pitch application, i.e., rapid table movement. Consequently, image quality at high spatial resolution and large pitch is becoming more depended on the flying spot technology, which provides a quasi-instant doubling of the in plane sampling rate.

IV. PITCH FACTOR, TABLE SPEED AND FEED

For spiral scans, the table feed D in mm per 360 degree rotations has to be chosen as a scan parameter. For single slice scanners with a gantry rotation time of 1 s, this corresponds exactly to the table speed d´ in mm/s. For scanners with variable rotation times this relation has to be modified. More importantly, the number M of simultaneously scanned slices has to be taken into account. The ratio of table feed D to total slice collimation MαS is generally termed the pitch or pitch factor:

$$P = \frac{D}{M \times S}$$

P = pitch (dimensionless)
D = table feed per rotation (mm/360 degree)
M = number of simultaneously scanned slices (1/360 degree)
S = nominal slice width (mm)

For a four–slice CT scanner, i.e. M = 4, with a nominal slice width of S = 1 mm and a table feed of D = 6 mm per rotation, for example, a pitch of P = 1.5 results.

The choice of the pitch factor is mostly determined by practical considerations – in general by the equation of which examination time T (s) is desirable or still acceptable for a given scan range R (mm). The desired table speed d´ = R/T (mm/s) then results directly. Taking the selected slice width and pitch factor into account, the table speed actually set is equally given by

$$d' = \frac{P \times M \times S}{T_{rot}}$$

d´ = table speed (mm/s)
p = pitch (dimensionless)

M = number of simultaneously scanned slices (1/360 degree).

S = nominal slice width

T_{rot} = rotation time

With the single slice helical CT the dimensionless term "pitch factor "was defined by the equation.

$$\text{Pitch factor} = \frac{\text{Table feed per 360 degree rotation}}{\text{Nominal slice width}}$$

For the multislice helical CT two descriptions of the pitch factor exist next to each other. The first definition supported by the CT manufactures is scientifically incorrect and results in higher pitch values by using the thickness of the single detector row collimation while the scientifically correct second definition describes the thickness of all irradiated detector rows. The resulting equations are:

1. $$\text{Pitch factor} = \frac{\text{Table feed per 360 degree rotation}}{\text{Thickness of a single detector row}}$$

2. $$\text{Pitch} = \frac{\text{Table feed per 360 degree rotation}}{\text{Nominal slice width} \times \text{Number of simultaneously acquired slices}}$$

V. GANTRY ROTATION, SCAN SPEED AND NUMBER OF SLICES

All manufactures agree that faster gantry rotation time less than 0.5 s are possible. However, the time reduction will be moderate due to the centrifugal powers by rotating the large and heavy gantry. Most engineers expect gantry rotation time of about 0.3 s in the future but a further increase of rotation speed will be extremely difficult to obtain with the known helical CT technology. Partial scans, sampling only a fraction of the data achieved during a 360 degree rotation, allow an image reconstruction of data obtained within a cardiac cycle which prevents pulsation artifacts. This is possible by new image reconstruction tools and allows sufficient cardiac scanning with multislice helical CT. The already available detector technology allows at least in theory the acquisition of more than 16 slices per gantry rotation. The matrix and hybrid detectors with more than 16 rows would theoretically allow the acquisition of more than 16 equally sized slices per gantry rotation. Some manufactures presented laboratory research with detectors allowing up to 256 slices per gantry rotation. All CT manufactures work on area detectors without any detector rows with a considerable higher quantum efficiency similar to the developments in conventional radiography.

VI. SLICE THICKNESS

The reconstructed slice thickness is dependent on the actually used detector configuration. If a slice thickness of 1 mm needs to be calculated the detector configuration has to be 4 × 1 mm or less. Then, the primary slice thickness being reconstructed in the clinical routine can be 1 mm or higher. It also allows the initial calculation of a slice thickness of 5 mm in order to reduce image noise or limit the number of images to be reviewed and archived. As long as the raw data is accessible the retrospectively calculated slice thickness can be reduced to 1 mm if it is required for any reason. When a detector configuration of 4 × 2 mm is chosen the smallest achievable slice thickness will be of course 2 mm.

VII. RECONSTRUCTION INCREMENT

The increment of the reconstruction (RI), i.e. the distance between the position of the neighboring imaging planes, is of great importance. The reconstruction of overlapping images brings fundamental advantages with regard to 3D spatial resolution and also diagnostic reliability. A 50% overlap, that is reconstruction increment of half a slice thickness, is a good value for orientation in spiral CT (RI = S/2), i.e., two images per slice thickness corresponds to sequential CT and does not utilize the special advantage of spiral CT. A strongly pronounced overlapping is (e.g. RI = S/3 or 67% overlap) advantageous for high 3D spatial resolution and for excellent MPR and 3D images.

VIII. IMAGE QUALITY

In general the slice sensitivity profiles of the multislice CT are similar to the single slice CT if the same scan parameters are used. However, the faster acquisition time of the multislice CT enables the operator to use much smaller slice thickness and/or decreased pitch factors which lead to significantly narrower slice sensitivity profiles. The resulting better spatial resolution enhances the image quality. Image quality in multislice CT must be optimised with respect to several factors. :

- The narrowest collimation, consistent with the coverage of a certain volume and with a certain scan time, to minimize partial volume effects and to optimize image quality.
- Fastest rotation time to maximize Z-coverage and to minimize motion blurring.
- Pitch of greater than 4 to preserve temporal resolution and minimize motion blurring.
- The exploitation of flying focal spot technology to avoid artifacts at high spatial resolution.

Anatomical structures that generate spiral artifacts are well known from single slice spirals. The most difficult situations arise from bony structures which are strongly inhomogeneous in axial direction. A demanding example is the base of the skull with bony structures abruptly ending in an image plane. Phantom studies have shown that a larger pitch and narrower collimation is much more favorable for suppressing artifacts than a lower pitch and wider collimation for equal Z-coverage. From image quality reasons only, the strength of multi-slice spiral scanning is the ability to cover anatomical volumes with narrowest collimation and thereby to minimize partial volume effects. This is only a matter of scanning technique (collimation) and is independent of the selected slice width. For optimization of image quality we derive the rule: the narrowest collimation should be selected which is consistent with volume coverage and scan time. This generally results in large pitch values, which helps to avoid motion blurring.

IX. MSCT SCAN PARAMETERS

For a proper and reproducible description of multislice CT scan parameters some factors have to be considered:

1. **Gantry rotation time** in seconds for a complete 360 degree rotation.
2. **Detector configuration** which describes the number of simultaneously acquired slices per gantry rotation and the width of the electronically combined detector elements (e.g. 4 × 1 mm).
3. **Reconstructed slice thickness** in mm which can be retrospectively calculated if the raw data set is still available. This can be done if the primary slice thickness is chosen as 1 mm for multiplanar reconstruction purposes but for the film or monitor reading a larger slice thickness resulting in considerably fewer images is still sufficient. However, the reconstructed slice thickness can only be larger or equal but never be smaller than the chosen detector configuration.
4. **Table speed** in mm per 360 degree gantry rotation.
5. **Pitch factor** is a dimensionless value defined by the equation pitch factor = table feed per 360 degree rotation/number of simultaneously acquired slices × normal slice width.
6. **Reconstruction interval** in mm for reducing volume averaging and improving multiplanar reconstruction.
7. **Tube current** in mA
8. **Tube voltage** in kV.

X. RADIATION EXPOSURE

Theoretically most vendors expect the radiation exposure to be decreased with multislice CT compared to single slice CT if the same scan parameters are used. In practice some manufactures still have hard or software problems leading to unchanged or even slightly higher radiation exposures. These shortcomings will probably be overcome in the near future by most vendors.

The major concern for radiation exposure will be driven by the advantages of the technique. The ability to scan during multiple perfusion phases after contrast material administration with thin slice thickness can lead to higher radiation exposures. Therefore the scan protocols should be individually adapted to the specific indication. Multislice helical CT requires further research in the future so that the optimum protocol for each individual patient is performed but not the optimum technique possible.

XI. CLINICAL APPLICATIONS

The advantage of MSCT is important to many applications of CT scanning, including survey exams in oncologic or trauma patients and the characterization of focal lung and liver lesions through the creation of thin sections respectively. However, the greatest impact has been on CT angiography, cardiac imaging, virtual endoscopy, and high-resolution imaging.

Those which really benefit from multislice CT include:

Trauma	: Larger single scan volumes in a single scan.
Paediatric	: Faster imaging reduces sedation.
Colonic screening	: Reduces respiratory artifacts, more optimal distension.
Lung screening	: Reduced respiratory artifacts, thin and thick slices from single scan.
Angiography	: Fast scanning ensures best use of contrast. Good z-axis resolution allows imaging of narrow vessels.
3D imaging	: Large number of narrow slices can provide high quality volume rendering.
Cardiac scanning	: Heart motion reduces quality of cardiac CT images.

Previous solution was EBCT scan time 0.1 s. Fast scan in MSCT can produce 180 degree scan in 0.3 s. Scan can be triggered by ECG signal to ensure minimum cardiac motion.

Coronary angiography. Non-invasive viewing of coronary arteries.

Visualisation of stenosis and soft plaque. Poor for vessels <1.5 mm diameter. Cardiac calcification scoring is easy.

CT Angiography

A fundamental advantage of a multislice scanner over monoslice systems is its ability to obtain a first circulation study of a rapidly injected contrast bolus with thinner images. Determining circulation time either by a preliminary minibolus or by online bolus tracking software is important in matching the acquisition interval to the first-circulation time of the injected bolus. As a result of the shorter acquisition time, the contrast used can be significantly reduced. CT angiography of the intracranial vessels benefits from the quick and detailed scanning technology of MSCT. At 1 mm collimation, the circle of Willis can be scanned within 10 sec. This permits the entire scan to be completed during the first pass of iodinated contrast material through the arterial system. The use of MSCT with CT angiography demonstrates the spatial relationship of an aneurysm with the feeding vessel, as well as the shape of the aneurysm itself, because the same bolus can be followed continuously throughout its course.

For CT angiography of the thoracoabdominal aorta a collimation of 2.5 mm and table feed of 5 mm at a rotation speed of 0.5 s is used. Volume coverage is from the thoracic inlet to the inguinal region, a 50 to 55-cm area that can be covered in an acquisition interval of approx. 20 sec. Reconstructions with 50% overlap are used, generating 400-450 images for the three-dimensional data set. A complete lower extremity study can be performed from the level of the renal vascular pedicles to the ankles. A 2.5 mm collimation, a pitch of 6 and 50% overlap reconstruction are used. A first-pass circulation study can be obtained without venous overlay. The total number of images generated is 800 to 1000. With multislice CT operating at pitch 6 and collimation of 4 × 1 mm, a CTA of the pulmonary arteries can be acquired in less than 25 sec. Image thickness of 1.25 mm significantly increases delectability of sub-segmental emboli in comparison to monoslice spiral CT using 2 to 3 mm image thickness. CTA of the visceral branch vessels can be performed significantly faster and/or with increased spatial resolution using a collimation of 1 mm allows for detection of even minor branches. The ability to cover the entire chest in 10 secs allows the scanning of children without sedation. This can be used to easily perform CTA of the large thoracic vessels before or after surgery of complex malformation.

High resolution imaging

Imaging of the temporal bone is a major challenge for clinical CT and a good example for the need for high resolution CT. Imaging of the temporal bone is improved using MSCT because the in-plane resolution can be greatly increased. The temporal bone is a structure of high intrinsic contrast and is routinely scanned with thin collimation. Both the 2 × 0.5 mm and the 4 × 1 mm mode on the somatom volume zoom are applicable (pitch 2 or 3. 5) and the tube current can be reduced to below 200 mAs. The reconstruction kernels enable maximum spatial resolution up to 24 line pairs per cm. At this resolution, the delicate structures of the middle and inner ear are sharply delineated and even subtle changes can be assessed. Another advantage of using MSCT to image the temporal bone is that the slice thickness is reduced to 1mm or below, thus minimizing the partial volume effects and further increasing image quality of subtle structures.

XII. ADVANTAGES OF MSCT OVER SINGLE SLICE

Advantages of multislice over single slice.

- Same acquisition in shorter time or
- Thin slice give better z-axis resolution or
- Scan larger volumes in the same time.
- Reduced artifacts
- Improved z-axis resolution
- New applications possible
- Existing applications have been improved or expanded
- More information available for radiologists
- Increased coverage per rotation
- Reduced overall tube loading
- Better use of contrast agents
- Greater coverage per breath hold

XIII. IMPACT ON RADIOLOGICAL PRACTICE

The large number of images generated by MSCT is a major issue for workstation performance, film display, and PACS archiving. The images should be previewed in a cine-paging format at a workstation for diagnostic purposes. Film hard copy will only be used for reference display. Planning for PACS must take into account this exponential growth in image data generated by this new technology. Rapid generation of 3D data sets is important for inclusion in the diagnostic study interpretation and for demonstration to referring clinicians. The hundreds or thousands of thin sections acquired using MSCT are incompatible with traditional viewing practice, thus MSCT will force a rapid transition of radiology from 2D to volumetric imaging.

CHAPTER 21

CT Imaging in CSF Leak

1. INTRODUCTION

Cerebrospinal fluid fistula has always been a diagnostic challenge. It is imperative to accurately localize the site of CSF fistula whenever surgical intervention is considered. Accurate localization increases the chance of successful preoperative identification of the site of CSF fistula and dural repairs. This eliminates the chance of negative or recurrence in exploration. Accurate preoperative localization has especially become important due to the emergence of newer minimally invasive surgical techniques using nasal endoscopes for the treatment of CSF fistula where the field of view is limited. Numerous techniques including plane skull radiography, tomography, intraoperative injection of fluorescein dye, positive contrast studies and radionuclide cisternography are all helpful in a limited way. For over a decade now, CT cisternography (CTC) has been considered the most reliable and accurate method in the diagnosis of CSF fistula. However CTC is invasive, time consuming and is contraindicated in patients with active meningitis. HRCT is highly effective in the demonstration of small bone defects at the site of CSF fistula.

2. TECHNIQUE

HRCT : 3 mm thin contiguous coronal sections are obtained through the floor of anterior cranial fossa, roof of the sphenoidal sinus and temporal bones in the prone position. Additional 1-1.5 mm thin contiguous sections are obtained through the region of interest. A field of view of 12 cm and a matrix of 512 × 512 are usually used. Axial sections can be obtained when there is CSF leakage suspected at the temporal bones. A bone algorithm is useful for greater bone detail.

CTC : Pledgets are placed in the areas most likely to detect a leak i.e. the pledgets may be placed high in the nasal cavity by the ENT surgeon. With all precautionary measures a lumbar puncture is done and suitable contrast material in instilled in the subarachnoid space. With suitable positioning contrast material is made to flow into the cranial subarachnoid space. The patient is placed in the position that clinically is related to the CSF leak and further imaging is done. Images are carefully studied for evidence of contrast material in the concerned region. This procedure is unlikely to be successful unless the patient is actively leaking at the time of study.

3. DIAGNOSIS

The imaging criteria for CSF leakage includes :

1. A bone defect,
2. CSF column extending across the bone defect extracranially
3. Herniation of brain/meninges across a bone defect or with air communicating from the paranasal sinuses intracranially.
4. On CT cisternography a contrast column extending from intracranial compartment would be diagnostic of CSF fistula.

4. DISCUSSION

For over a decade, contrast CTC has been considered the gold standard for the diagnosis of CSF fistula. CTC has a high true positive rate reaching 92% in active and 40% in inactive CSF leaks. However CTC is invasive, time consuming, slightly uncomfortable and carries a small risk of complications such as infection and headache. CTC is relatively contraindicated in patients with active meningitis and raised intracranial pressure. Over the last decade there has been lot of advances in CT technology. This has resulted in better quality images; thinner slices (up to 1 mm) with high spatial resolution are possible with a modern CT scanner with a much shorter span of time. Though the most probable site of CSF fistula is found in the floor of anterior cranial fossa predominantly in the cribriform plate and/or fovea ethmoidalis (roof of the ethmoidal sinus) or the roof of the sphenoidal sinus or the tegmen tympani (roof of the middle ear cavity of the temporal bone), fistulas may be seen at the lateral wall of the internal auditory canal. In the absence of demonstration of CSF fistula at the floor of anterior cranial fossa, roof of the sphenoid sinus or tegmen tympani of the temporal bone, the lateral wall of the internal auditory canal should be looked for carefully especially in patients with bilateral CSF leakage and unilateral deafness.

5. SCAN PROTOCOL

HRCT should be the first line of investigation in patients diagnosed as CSF rhinorrhea with clinical or by laboratory methods. MRI cisternography may be performed if the findings of the HRCT are equivocal. If either of these modalities fails to convincingly show the site of fistula CTC can be performed, as a last resort possibly with a nasal pledget as the leakage could be extremely slow to be detected on a routine study.

CHAPTER

22

CT-Guided Radiotherapy Planning

1. INTRODUCTION

There is considerable variation in the extent to which CT is used for radiotherapy planning. It is unlikely that many intracranial, intrathoracic and intra-abdominal lesions are now treated without a diagnostic CT (or MRI) images to show the extent of disease. The axial information about the size of the lesion and its relation to other organs, in general terms, can be used by the therapist in the planning procedure. However, in many centres only a minority of patients proceed to have a formal planning CT examination to allow direct treatment planning from the electronic CT data. But this is likely to change rapidly in the near future as radiotherapy departments replace some of their conventional simulators with low-cost CT units specifically designed for radiotherapy planning.

2. ADVANTAGES

There are considerable advantages in using the direct CT data for therapy planning. Firstly an accurate surface outline of the torso is obtained. The lesion can be accurately related to this outline. Furthermore, for some forms of radiation used for treatment, the attenuation by the tissues is very similar to that in the original CT data acquisition. Thus the attenuation values can be used directly for planning purposes. Most manufacturers have sophisticated computed planning packages which allow the isodose contours to be displayed on the CT image. As such work is labour-intensive, and because the radiotherapist often tries out several options, it is usual to have this facility on a stand-alone system so that the main evolution console is not blocked.

3. TECHNIQUE

With increasingly sophisticated imaging, radiotherapy planning is also becoming increasingly complex. It is now possible to highlight a lesion and to demonstrate it in a 3D image. Such 3D work for intracranial lesions is becoming routine in some centers, both for neurosurgical and radiotherapeutic approaches. It is important to realize that there are several differences in techniques between CT examinations performed for diagnostic and for planning purposes. For diagnostic studies, respiration is suspended, bowel loops are opacified by contrast medium and the image is often expanded so that the key organs are optimally demonstrated. For planning studies, after the coordinates ***x, y*** and ***z*** have been precisely located and the skin of the patient has been appropriately marked, the images are obtained in a rather different manner. No specific instructions about respiration are given; during the subsequent radiotherapy the patient breathes at will. The images are obtained without magnifications so that the white skin circumference is visible. Ideally the bowel is not opacified; the presence of contrast medium upsets subsequent planning based on measurement attenuation, although some software systems can allow for this.

4. SCOPE OF THE TECHNIQUE

Planning CT examinations may be performed in various positions (e.g. prone) and with various other manoeuvres (e.g. with the bladder full for a prostate neoplasm). Despite the increasing sophistication of CT planning techniques, there is scant evidence of improved cure rates brought about through these measures. Perhaps the best that can be hoped for is that the morbidity of radiotherapy is reduced. And, indeed, it has been shown that the use of CT planning techniques can reduce the side-effects of radiotherapy by reducing the dose to critical organs adjacent to the lesion (e.g. a lower rectal dose and fewer associated symptoms when treating pelvis neoplasms).

CHAPTER 23

CT-Guided Stereotaxy and Gamma Knife Surgery

1. INTRODUCTION

Routine neurosurgical procedures are associated with high morbidity and mortality, as the brain tissue tolerates retraction and displacement poorly. In the last two decades there has been a major progress in the development of newer minimally invasive surgical procedures, which are safer and highly precise. Stereotactic and gamma knife surgery are amongst some of these minimally invasive neurosurgical procedures. The introduction of newer imaging modalities such as CT has played a very important role in further improving surgical skills. Surgery for deep parts of the brain such as the basal ganglia and thalami involves an unavoidable and unacceptable risk of damage to important areas lying superficial to or adjacent to these regions. Thus, conventional open surgical technique is an essentially inappropriate method to use for operations in the depths of the brain, irrespective of the sophistication of modern microsurgical techniques. The availability of the precise 3D database provided by CT brought revolution in stereotactic surgery.

2. STEREOTAXY

Principles of Stereotaxy

The aim of the techniques is to relate the location of deep and inaccessible intracerebral structures to a three-dimensional cartesian axis system. The first step in this process is to enclose the head in such a system which is done by fixing rigid metal frame. The borders of the frame then constitute the cartesian axis, while the cranium serves as a platform to support the frame and the cerebrum is enclosed both physically and conceptually within a microcosm, where every point can be precisely defined in space. Thus it is possible to define any intracranial target with respect to the frame. However, to be of any use, the frame itself must be a platform for a device, which will hold an instrument or electrode, to be introduced in to the brain, to reach the target. The smaller diameter of the instrument used and the mechanical stability with which they are held and introduced by means of a rigid holder and guide and the extreme accuracy of the localization implicit in the method are the basis of the exceptionally atraumatic nature of stereotactic procedures.

A great variety of different stereotactic system has been designed over the last 40 years. The Lekesell stereotactic system was the first to be constructed with a view to ease of application and frequent use. The instrument holder is mounted on the arc and move transversely across the whole circumference of the arc. When the axis values for the target point have been determined, the center of the arc will always coincide with this target point. This arrangement allows a needle to be pointed at its target from an almost infinite number of directions. An important point of the design is that, for a given target setting, the point of the instrument introduced to the center of the arc does not move.

The development of CT has greatly facilitated stereotactic procedures. These techniques render space-occupying lesion truly visible and thus simple to localize. Moreover the modern machine can incorporate software, which will superimpose a stereotactic grid on the film, and this makes localization extremely simple. This use of the stereotactic frame with CT unit necessitated the development of an adapter to fix the stereotactic frame to the CT table, to ensure that the axis system of the frame and the axis system of the CT software were concordant.

3. INDICATIONS AND CONTRAINDICATIONS

Stereotaxy is not to be considered as alternative to other forms of treatment but is to be used in addition to the more traditional armamentarium of neurosurgical options. Stereotactic biopsies are usually performed in intraaxial lesions which are deep-seated and not suitable for conventional craniotomy. Subcortical, centrally located, basal ganglia, thalamic, brain stem or deep cerebellar tumours can be biopsied easily and safely by CT stereotaxy. CT stereotaxy is a preferred method for obtaining biopsies in non-enhancing hypodense lesion which are usually infiltrative tumours. Patient with large mass effect have risk of herniation of brain parenchyma. Vascular malformation can have a risk of intracranial hemorrhage. Pituitary stalk lesions, near the circle of Willis, have risk of vascular damage.

4. TECHNIQUE

A stereotactic frame is fixed to the head of the patient usually under local anesthesia. The frame consists of radiopaque indicator plates known as fiducial lines. The target can be placed in the center of the frame. Subsequently, the patient is transferred to the CT examination table. Scans are obtained through the axial plane without any tilt in the patient position. The fiducial lines are seen as dots in the CT image. The frame center is found by drawing diagonals from the opposite vertical fiducial line to each other. Where these lines cross is the center of the frame. The X and Y values at this point are 100 for both. Thereafter a grid centered at the center of the frame is superimposed. These fiducial lines are in the form of a backwards-N . An extra vertical line at the front on one indicates the orientation. Because the oblique fiducial line (a) is drawn at a 45 angle to vertical (b) fiducial line, a = b. Because a = b, it is possible to assess the "Z" value for given CT slice, by measuring the distance b. The b distance can be measured from the CT images (i.e. the distance between the oblique and posterior fiducials), and the Z value is determined. "Z" ="b" + 40 because the posterior vertical fiducial line is at 40 on the "Y" axis. After all the calculations are made, the planning is done preoperatively and after mechanical adjustments on the stereotactic frames, the approaching angular settings are done. The biopsy probe is inserted through a burr hole and directed by means of a stereotactic instrument through the lesion in question. An approach must be planned which avoids all vascular structures and provides the best sampling of the lesion.

5. SURGICAL APPROACH

For subcortical lesion anterior to the rolantic fissure the approach is anterior to posterior. Lesion posterior to central sulcus is approached from the posterior trajectory. Subinsular lesion is approached from a coronal entry point. Pulvinar lesion is approached from posterior parietal point. It is essential to plan a biopsy trajectory parallel to the CT slices.

CT-GUIDED GAMMA KNIFE SURGERY

I. INTRODUCTION

Gamma knife treatment is considered to be the most sophisticated tool in the minimal invasive neurosurgery. It is a powerful neurosurgical tool with a very high (submillimeter) degree of accuracy for treating intracranial brain lesions and vascular malformations (AVMs), which are inaccessible to conventional surgical procedures or are located in close proximity to neurocritical or neuroeloquent structures. Radiosurgery is devised as a procedure whereby a single high dose of radiation is delivered to a small and critically located intracranial volume without opening the skull. The gamma knife is not really a knife at all but rather a curved steel helmet comprising of 201 individual cobalt 60 sources fixed mechanically over the interior of a hemisphere resembling a large bowl which fits over the patient head. The narrow gamma beams are directed through the ports of collimator helmet to intersect at a target in the brain. The variable size together with submillimeter positioning accuracy achieved with the Lekesell stereotactic frames to produce extremely well directed radiation to any location deep inside the brain. The exquisite precision of the radiation field administered at a single stage is similar to any neurosurgical procedure and hence the tool was named a "knife". Since gamma ray from cobalt 60 were the source of radiation, this neurosurgical tool was called the "gamma knife". These gamma rays may be viewed as high-energy beams that can be focused in much the same way as a magnifying glass focuses sun beam. The sub-millimeter accuracy and lack of mobile parts in the Lekesell gamma knife (LGK) provide enhanced safety, reproducibility and reliability. Gamma knife radiosurgery can be an adjunct or alternative to open microneurosurgery. Small to medium sized AVMs are the best indication for primary GK treatment

TREATMENT PROCEDURE

A frame called the Lekesell frame is fixed to the head of the patient usually under local anesthesia. After the frame is fixed, the patient is taken to the radiology department for CT. It provides the visualization and accurate localization of the target in the X, Y, and Z-axis after which the patient is moved to a resting area. CT is useful to cross check accuracy and to evaluate the adjacent bones. High resolution (512 × 512 matrix) 1 mm contiguous images are obtained after intravenous contrast administration. Absolute care is taken to avoid image distortion. A spirit level is used to avoid a tilt. The distance between the anterior and posterior fiducial is measured on both the sides so that the measured value does not differ by more than 1 mm. In critical areas or targets anywhere near the visual pathways, images of these vital structures are also included.

The image obtained in the radiology department is then transferred to a computer workstation. On this computer, the target is defined by keeping in mind the critical structures of the brain. Planning is done so as to treat the lesion effectively without damaging critical structures of the brain. Obvious single or multiple set of doses are placed on the lesion in two-dimensional and three-dimensional use to achieve a dose distribution which matches the geometry of the lesion.

Once the dose planning is done, the patient is moved on to the GK couch with the head within one of the four helmets. The frame is used to position the head at the focal point of the cobalt 60 beams.

CHAPTER

24

IV Iodinated Contrast Media

1. IODINE

Water soluable contrast media are compounds containing iodine. Intravascular iodinated contrast media were introduced into clinical practice in 1928 by Moses Swick. Atomic weight of iodine is 127. The daily iodine turnover is about .0001 grams (.1 mg) and total body iodine is .01 grams (10 mg). Iodine attenuates X-ray very much because of its high atomic number. The substances other than iodine do not offer contrast; they act as carrier and increase solubility, and decrease toxicity.

2. BIOCHEMISTRY

Today's contrast medicines are derived from triiodinated benzene rings that carry an acid group—COOH at carbon No. 1 and three iodine atoms at carbon 2, 4 and 6. In position 3 and 5 other substituents can be added and these influence the behavior of contrast media to a large extent. Since they have to be dissolved in high concentration their salts are used. Usually Na or meglumine cations are used to prepare salts of contrast medicines. So Na or meglumine salts are very soluble, to be dissolved in high concentrations if required. But when they are dissolved, they dissociate into two particles—cation and anion. The anion is actually the particle responsible for the contrast. The type of contrast media, which dissociates into ions when in solution, is called Ionic Contrast media (ICM).

Ionic contrast media may cause problems because they have a high osmolality and also they carry electrical charges. The C_3 and C_5 side chains (radicals) are substituted amines of NH_2, which reduce toxicity and promote solubility. Proprietary brands differ only in minor modification of R3 and R5. Major drawback of conventional ionic contrast media is high osmolality. Ideal

Ionic monomer

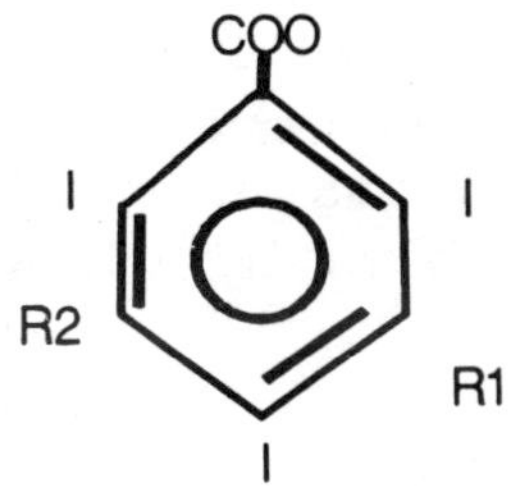

Tri-iodinated benzene ring

contrast media is without any nonradiopaque cations, which serves only as a carrier. Radiopacity depends on number of iodine atoms in each molecule of contrast media. High radiopacity and low osmolality are the desirable requirements. Osmolality is number of particles per kilogram of solute and osmolarity is number of particles per litre of solution. Blood osmolality is the order of 300 mOsm/kg. Ionic contrast medium has up to1800 mOsm/kg. The non-ionic monomers are usually 600-700 mOsm/kg which still is about twice the osmolality of blood. The non-ionic dimer iotrolan has about 300 mOsm/kg making it iso-osmolar (isotonic).

Iodine particle ratio = Number of iodine per molecule/number of particles of solute in solution per molecule.

Constituents other than contrast media

1) Buffers : Stabilize the contrast medium solution in a particular pH range.
2) Chelating agents : They bind heavy metal ions, which may get into the solution during the manufacturing process or come from contrast media bottle wall.

Contrast media viscosity

Viscosity influences injectability. Besides weight, size, shape and concentration of contrast medium molecule, temperature also determines viscosity. Warming of contrast media to body temperature may decrease this viscosity dramatically.

3. METHODS TO REDUCE OSMOLALITY

Three different ways to reduce contrast media osmolality were developed.

1) Method I

Coupling of benzene rings making an ionic dimer or trimer. It has lower osmolality, but still carries electrical charge. Iodine particle ratio is 3 : 1.

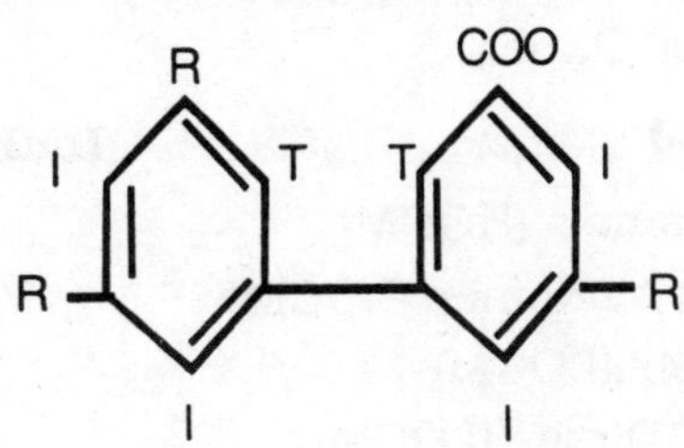

Ionic dimer

2) Method II

Replacing the acid group with a compound that no longer dissociates into ions but still is soluble enough to provide enough contrast.

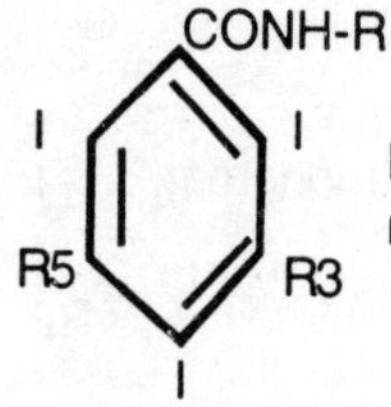

Non-ionic monomer

3) Method III

A combination of both these processes leads to the non-ionic dimer which is an iso-osmolal non-ionic dimer.

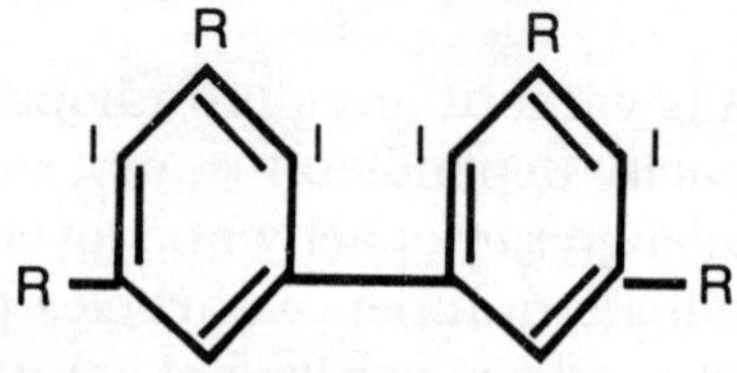

Non-ionic dimer

4. CLASSIFICATION

A. Classification by osmolality

1) High osmolar
   Iopthalmate metrizoate 3:2
   Diatrizoate
2) Low osmolar
   I) Non-ionic monomer 3:1
      Iohexol, Iopromide, Iopamidol, Ioversol
   ii) Dimeric (ionic) 3:1
      Ioglycomate, Iocarmate
   iii) Non-ionic dimmer 6:1
      Iotrolan

B. Classification by ionicity

1) Ionic contrast media
   a) Monomeric (High osmolar)
      Iopthalmate, Diatrizoate, metrizoate
   b) Dimeric (Low osmolar)
      Glycermate, Iocermate
2) Non-ionic
   a) Monomer - Iohexol, Iopromode, iopamidol
   b) Dimer.

Compound	Iodine Atom : Particle Ratio	Osmolality
Ionic Monomer (HOCM)	3 : 2	1500
Non-ionic Monomer (LOCM)	3 : 1	600
Ionic Dimer (LOCM)	6 : 2	560
Non-ionic Dimer (LOCM)	6 : 1	300

5. CONTRAST MEDIA AND ORGANS

Kidney

Contrast media is excreted by glomerular filteration. Under normal circumstances there is neither active contrast media secretion nor reabsorption by the kidneys. On the way to pelvicalyceal system the urine becomes more concentrated in the kidney by means of water absorption. Because water is reabsorbed, the concentrations of the various substances in the urine increase including contrast media. So the contrast medium becomes more and more concentrated. However the contrast media itself binds to some fluid so it also acts like an osmotic diuretic. Non-ionic contrast media are more concentrated in urine than ionic contrast media. It also depends on the cation used. Sodium salts become more concentrated than meglumine salts, because sodium can be reabsorbed. When reabsorbed the sodium carries with it a certain amount of water which otherwise would have remained in the urine.

Heart

Contrast media may have many different effects upon the heart muscle cells as well as the conducting system. Myocardial contractility and cardiac system may be altered, Pressure load and volume load increased. All the effects are much less pronounced and less frequent with the injection of non-ionic contrast media.

Vessels

Contrast media affect arteries and veins by their osmolality and also by chemotoxicity. With arterial injection a peripheral vasodilatation may result. This is more pronounced with increasing osmolality and may be directly involved in pain production. Compensatory increase in cardiac output maintains the blood pressure. Endothelial damages are more in veins than arteries. Here the contrast media is not carried away and diluted as fast as with arterial injections. The longer the contrast media can act on the endothelium, the more pronounced are the resulting change.

Brain

The neurogenic complications with contrast media occur only when they cross blood-brain barrier, they cause problems like convulsion. The problems are more with ionic contrast media.

Thyroid

Contrast media can affect the thyroid even though the iodine is bound very tightly to contrast media molecule. Contrast media contain minimum amounts of iodide and iodide also splits off the contrast media molecule by enzymatic action in the body. In the presence of autonomous cells in the thyroid this iodide which is taken up by thyroid cells may lead to an increased and uncontrolled hormone production. To a certain extent this increased production may be balanced by a decrease in hormone production by the normal cells of the gland. However if a certain level is exceeded symptoms of thyroid hyperfunction may result.

6. SIDE EFFECTS

Contrast media side effects can be caused by different mechanisms. Some of them are still unknown or subject to debate. However a number of influencing factors have been identified.

(1) Some effects are due to the electrical charge of contrast media (that is why non-ionic is better tolerated than ionic).

(2) Side effects are more pronounced and frequent with an increase in osmolality, protein binding and lipophilicity.

(3) Hydrophilicity decreases side effects.

There is no single theory to explain all the adverse reactions that could be encountered. The side effects caused by the above three factors are dose dependent. There are number of reactions, which are non-dose dependent and caused by other mechanisms. Many of them look like clinical manifestations of allergic reactions like itching, bronchospasm etc. Histamine, the typical allergy substance, has been shown to be responsible for a number of these problems. Since in many of the cases the signs and symptoms nonetheless resemble allergies these reactions are called pseudoallergic or allergoid reaction. Severe reaction after contrast media resembles those of anaphylactic reaction caused by allergic process.

Effects on Cardiovascular System

1) Cardiac contractility : Ionic contrast causes a decrease in contractility followed by an increase in contractility.
2) Coronary perfusion increases.
3) Conduction time is delayed. Increase PR and QRS Complex
4) Dysarrhythmia.
5) Peripheral vessels/Vasodilatation may occur. Pain and warmth due to hyper osmolality.
6) Endothelial damage.
7) Inhibit coagulation.

Effects on Central Nervous System

If hyperosmolar solutions are used opening of blood-brain barrier may result. Blood-brain barrier is reestablished within a few minutes to two hours after these injections. Contrast media can have direct neurotoxic effect when it is in direct contact with nerve cells or brain tissue, that is defective blood-brain barrier, during myelography etc. Seizure and cortical blindness are the clinical manifestations. Under condition with reduced cerebral flow, the contact time of the contrast media and consequently the risk for blood-brain barrier damage is increased. In such conditions the least irritating contrast media should be used e.g. subarachnoid haemorrhage.

Nephrotoxicity

Contrast medium induced renal failure is defined as rise in serum creatinine level of at least 1 mg/dl within 48 hours after contrast medium administration. It is accompanied by oliguria in about 3/4th of patients.

Causes

- Reduction in renal blood flow caused by contrast medium injection
- Direct toxic effects on the tubules
- Contrast medium may combine with urinary proteins to form semisolid plugs obstructing the tubular lumen. This is a probable explanation, which also explains prolonged nephrogram.

The Risk

Certain patients are at higher risk for contrast medium induced renal failure.

a) Dehydration : Dehydration causes increased concentration of contrast medium in urine, which cause damage to tubular lining. It also increases the time that tubular epithelium is exposed to this concentrated solution causing more damage.

b) Large amount of contrast media : Risk is higher when dose is more than .8 gram iodine/kg.

c) Pre-existing renal disease : If the number of functioning nephrons is reduced the ones still working will receive a larger contrast medium load. In addition if there is a concomitant proteinuria the risk for plug formation is increased. A serum creatinine <1.4 mg/dl is normal. Some old patients have reduced total muscle mass. So less creatinine is produced. If an old patient has a value of 1.4 mg this is considered as evidence of reduced renal function.

d) Diabetes mellitus : Patients with renal insufficiency and/or proteinuria are at particular risk. Contrast medium can exacerbate the nephrotoxicity and renal failure.

e) Paraproteinuria : Contrast medium causes plug formation.

f) CVS diseases : Vascular obstruction can cause decreased perfusion and kidney function.

g) Advanced age : > 70
h) Hypertension
i) Hyperuremia and use of diuretic.

Prevention of contrast media induced nephrotoxicity

i) Identify patient at risk
ii) Give least amount of contrast medium
iii) Hydrate well
iv) Loop diuretic

Upper limit of contrast medium dose

- Ionic contrast medium 2 ml/kg
- Nonionic contrast medium 5 ml/kg
- For cardiac catheterization 5 ml/kg/(mg × 300ml)/serum creatinine (Mg/dl)

7. ADVERSE REACTION

A. Idiosyncratic anaphylactic reaction

1) Most dreaded, frequent, serious and fatal
2) Usually begins within 5 minutes
3) Not dose dependent

Mechanisms

a) Inhibition of enzymes : Cholinesterase, which deactivates acetylcoline-esterase symptoms of vagal stimulation.
b) Release of vasoactive substances like : histamine and serotonin leading to vasomotor collapse.
c) Activation of physiological cascade system : Complement system, kinin system, fibrinolytic system.
d) Anxiety, apprehension.

B. Non-idiosyncratic dose dependent

a) Chemotoxic : May be related to toxicity of whole contrast media molecules rather than to iodinc content.
b) Osmotoxic (hyperosmolality related) :
   - RBC damage, endothelial damage
   - Blood brain barrier damage, Vasodilatation
   - Cardiac depression, Hypervolumia

c) Vasomotor reactions
d) Direct organ toxicity
e) Vagal reaction

8. RISK FOR ADVERSE REACTION

- Asthma - 5 times risk
- History of allergy - 4 times risk
- Previous adverse reaction to contrast medium - 11 times risk
- Age above 60
- Cardiac diseases 4 to 5 times

Premedication

Premedication does not eliminate the possibility of a subsequent reaction. All cases that had contrast medium reaction previously may not develop reaction next time. A change from ionic to nonionic is helpful. Even different types of nonionic contrast medium can be tried. Premedication in combination with the use of nonionic contrast medium further decreases the prevelance of subsequent reaction. In high risk patients premedication and use of nonionic contrast medium seems wise.

Prophylactive treatment Regime

- Prednisolone 40 mg orally, 13H, 7H and 1H, before IV contrast injection and Diphen hydramine 50 mg orally 1 hour before contrast injection; or
- Methylprednisole : 32 mg orally 12H, 2H, before contrast injection and Diphen hydramine 30 mg orally 1 hour before IV injection.

Remember tumour lysis syndrome may be induced by corticosteroids in certain patients (leukaemia, lymphoma); so they should be avoided. In patients with pheochromocytoma hypertensive crisis has been reported after contrast medium. The administration of an alpha adrenergic blocker in sufficient time prior to contrast medium have been suggested.

Factors predisposing to adverse reaction

- Previous adverse reaction (6-10 times)
- History of asthma/bronchospasm (5-10 times)
- History of allergy or atropy, cardiac disease (2-5 times)
- Dehydration, hematological or metabolical conditions
- Sickle cell disease, thrombotic tendency, multiple myeloma, pheochromocytoma
- Renal diseases, anxiety, apprehension

	Ionic	Nonionic
% of total reaction	12	3
% of severe reaction	0.2	0.04
% of very severe reaction	0.04	0.004

9. COMPLICATIONS

1) **Minor reaction—5-15% incidence :**
   - Flushing, nausea, arm pain, pruritis
   - Vomiting, headache, urticaria
2) **Intermediate reaction :**
   - Above reactions occur in higher severity
   - Moderate hypotension, bronchospasm
3) **Severe life-threatening reaction :**
   - Severe form of above reaction, convulsion, unconsciousness, laryngeal edema,
   - Severe bronchospasm, pulmonary edema, cardiovascular collapse

10. EXCRETION OF CONTRAST MEDIA

Normally about 30% of the contrast medium is excreted via the kidney in the first and almost 75% in six hours. The kidney excretes more than 95% of contrast medium. Extra renal routes called heterotropic or vicarious excretion are responsible for not more than about 5% of the contrast medium excretion under normal circumstances. In patients with impaired renal function, extra-renal contrast medium excretion is more pronounced approaching 10% of the injected dose.

11. FEW POINTS TO REMEMBER

Opened bottle

Should be used within 4 hours. Contamination is more with non-ionic contrast medium.

Storage of contrast medium

Should be stored at room temperature. Crystals may form if cooled to around 0°C. Crystals can be dissolved if heated to 80°C. If kept for long time at 300°C it promotes decomposition.

Disinfections

Ionic contrast media which contain more than 300 mg iodine/ml have antimicrobic activity. This is not due to the iodine but due to high osmolality and chemotoxicity.

Blood test after contrast medium injection

Thyroid tests are disturbed. Also uptake of radioactive tracers into thyroid is reduced for 2 to 6 weeks. Urine specific gravity increases after contrast medium injection. Urine protein may be increased. Electrolytes especially those of iron and copper may be disturbed. Blood urea, creatinine, bilirubin and cholesterol are influenced. Liver enzymes also may be affected.

Pregnancy

Contrast medium can enter fetal circulation. Also it is excreted through breast milk for 5 days.

Why nausea and vomiting

Area postrena the trigger zone for nausea and vomiting do not have a blood brain barrier and may be stimulated by contrast medium.

Delayed reaction

Delayed reaction after 4-6 hours reported in 4%.

Renal tract

Contrast is better with low osmolar contrast medium (less diuresis) compared to high osmolar contrast medium. There is very little difference in renal toxicity between low osmolar and high osmolar contrast media. But low osmolar contrast media is preferred in those with impaired renal function.

Nervous system

Low osmolar contrast media is preferred: If high osmolar contrast media are used meglumine salts are preferred.

Cardiovascular system

Low osmolar contrast media is preferred over high osmolar contrast media in peripheral angio. If ionic contrast media are used meglumine salts are preferred as they cause less vasodilatation.

CHAPTER 25

Contrast Enhancement Techniques

1. INJECTION ROUTE

The proximal forearm or antecubital vein is the best site for administration of contrast material. Indwelling central lines are not recommended for contrast injection. Many of these lines have a lower PSI rating than standard intravenous catheters. In some patients, central lines are damaged by the rapid injection of contrast material. If possible, a peripheral intravenous line should be started and used for the administration of contrast.

2. EXTRAVASATION

Because of the routine use of intravenous contrast material in the CT department, extravasation of contrast medium into the subcutaneous tissue sometimes occurs. The use of mechanical injectors produces the best results. However, if appropriate precautions are not taken, extravasation is likely to be more common and more severe with the routine use of a pressure injector. Every effort should be made to avoid contrast extravasation because the results may be serious. Most injuries involve small volumes and are not clinically significant. Slight swelling and erythema may develop and usually subside without complication. Severe tissue necrosis can be caused by even small volume (less than 10 ml) extravasation and surgical intervention may be required. There is no universally accepted treatment for contrast extravasation. Treatment may include local application of heat for the first 6 hours, then application of cold; local injection of isoproterenol or propranolol; local injection of steroids; and surgical drainage. The results of the various courses of treatment are mixed and the best method of reducing injury is prevention. Recent animal studies show that nonionic contrast medium is less injurious to cutaneous and subcutaneous tissue than conventional high-osmolar contrast material. Strict adherence to the following guidelines will substantially reduce the risk of contrast extravasation. Recent animal studies show that non-ionic contrast medium is less injurious to cutaneous and subcutaneous tissue than conventional high-osmolar contrast meterial :

1. Start an intravenous line with a 1.5 inch, 18 to 20 gauge needle with a flexible (plastic) cannula. A needle that is 22 gauge or smaller requires injection rate decreased.
2. Monitor the injection site, preferably an antecubital vein, during the initial phase of injection. Swelling at the site of injection indicates extravasation, and the injection should be stopped immediately.
3. Warm the contrast medium to body temperature to reduce contrast viscosity.
4. Do not use multiple injections into the same vein.

3. EFFECTS OF CONTRAST ON TISSUE ENHANCEMENT

Three phases of tissue enhancement are commonly discussed in CT: the bolus phase, the nonequilibrium phase, and the equilibrium phase. The difference between these phases is predominantly determined by the rate at which the contrast material is delivered at the time that elapses between injection and scanning. The bolus phase, which immediately follows an intravenous bolus injection, is characterized by an attenuation difference of 30 or more Hounsfield units (HU) between the aorta and the inferior vena cava. In the nonequilibrium phase, which follows the bolus phase, there is a difference of 10 to 30 HU between the aorta and the inferior vena cava. The last phase is the equilibrium phase, in which the attenuation difference is less than 10 HU. Compared with examinations performed before the administration of contrast medium, visualization of tumors in the liver is improved in the nonequilibrium phase, but not in the equilibrium phase. Scanning in the equilibrium phase does not improve visualization of hepatic tumors compared with precontrast examination.

4. ADMINISTRATION TECHNIQUES

Although the usefulness of intravenous contrast agents is universally accepted, there is little agreement as to the best method of administering contrast material. The two most common methods of administering contrast material are the drip infusion and bolus techniques. In the drip infusion technique, an intravenous line is initiated and contrast medium is allowed to drip in over a period of several minutes. Scanning usually begins after approximately 50 ml of contrast material is injected (roughly 2–3 minutes). The remaining contrast medium continues to drip until administration is complete. This method is not recommended because virtually all of the scans acquired with this technique are taken in the equilibrium phase. The bolus technique of contrast enhancement employs scanning after a rapid injection of contrast material. A volume of contrast of 50 to 100 ml is injected at a rate of 1 to 4 ml/sec shortly before scanning begins. The interval between the initiation of the injection and the start of scanning is critical, particularly in high speed scanning. The appropriate interval is also debated. When scanners cannot scan the entire area of interest rapidly, a modification of the bolus technique is used. This method, which is called dynamic sequential bolus CT, employs a series of smaller bolus injections given at intervals over the length of the scan procedure. Another injection protocol used in conjunction with older, slower scanners is biphasic injection. A bolus phase is used to gain peak enhancement, and a slower second phase is used to extend enhancement until the scanner can complete the study.

Injection Techniques For Spiral Scanning

In general, because of its increased speed, spiral scanning allows for a single bolus injection. This bolus is achieved with higher flow rates, and it increases the enhancement level for the entire study. Again, the interval between the injection of contrast material and scanning plays a critical role. Spiral CT because of its speed allows evaluation of the same organ in multiple phases of contrast enhancement. For example, liver can be scanned in three phases of contrast enhancement after a single bolus injection i.e. arterial, venous, and parenchymal (equilibrium) phases. This is called multiphasic study(Bi/triphasic). This procedure is extensively utilised in imaging for hepatic metastasis. Similarly kidneys can be scanned in different phases like vascular (arterial) 10-15 sec, cortical nephrographic 20-45 sec, parenchymal nephrographic 45-120 sec, and excretory 2-3 minutes. Depending on the pathology in mind the exact timing (phase) of renal study can be planned to provide the optimum information.

5. GASTROINTESTINAL CONTRAST MEDIUM

Barium Sulfate Solutions

Conventional Ba suspensions cannot be used in CT since they cause streak artifacts. Also simple dilution of the same preparation will not serve the purpose due to their tendency to settle after ingestion. Even though products containing 1-2% barium sulphate are manufactured specifically for CT they are not commonly used and not easily available in India. If it is used a minimum of 500 ml of 2% dilute barium sulphate should be given 45 minutes to 2 hours before scanning. An additional 200 ml should be given just before scanning to fill the stomach and proximal small bowel.

Water-Soluble Agents

1000-1500 ml of 2-3% solution of ionic contrast media are universally used for gastrointestinal opacification in CT examination. When rectosigmoid or any pelvic pathology is suspected, rectal administration of contrast material may be necessary. In these cases, 200 to 500 ml of a 1%-3% solutions are given by enema.

CHAPTER 26

CT-Guided Procedures

I. INTRODUCTION

CT is a valuable tool for use in interventional procedures such as biopsies and abscess drainage. The use of CT to guide percutaneous procedures offers several advantages. CT images provide precise three-dimensional localization of lesions and permit the radiologist to plan an access route to the lesion by showing the relation of the surrounding structures. Because the tip of the needle within the structure can be visualized, procedures can be performed even on very small lesions. Patients can be placed in a variety of positions to allow easier access to the lesion.

CT-guided procedures are most useful in the :

1. Retroperitoneum
2. Pelvis
3. Mediastinum
4. Small lesions or collections less than 3 cm in diameter
5. Masses located near major vascular structures
6. Intra-abdominal lesions surrounded by the loops of bowel.
7. Lesions that are not easily shown by either ultrasound or flouroscopy

In theory, the risk associated with needle biopsy increases as needle diameter increases. When a cutting needle is used, the risk is even greater. However the overall complication rate is small, approximately 2%. The primary complication of biopsy procedure is bleeding. Highly vascularised lesions increase the risk. A bleeding disorder is a contraindication to percutaneous biopsy. However, patients are often treated with blood products or medications to temporarily remedy the disorder so that the biopsy can be performed.

Biopsy can be performed on virtually any scanner. The purpose of CT-guided biopsy is to differentiate neoplastic disease from other processes, such as inflammatory disease, postoperative changes, post-therapeutic changes, or normal structures. Therefore, the goal in a biopsy procedure is to obtain an adequate sample for laboratory evaluation with minimal trauma or surrounding tissues. This goal is achieved with accurate and expedient placement of the needle.

II. ADVANTAGES OF CT-GUIDED PROCEDURES

- Accuracy of localization of lesion.
- Resolution could be less than 1 mm.
- Versatility.
- Proper selection of safest path.
- Choice of wide variety of instrument.

If the needle is placed within an anatomic area and the CT scan shows the needle in that area, then the needle must lie within the 10 mm section of the abdomen corresponding to the CT section. The ability to localize the needle tip consistently and accurately in an axial plane is a distinct advantage of CT over fluoroscopy or ultrasound. Versatility is still one of the most valuable advantages of CT-guided procedures. Since the skin is unimpeded, no "holding" devices are required. There is significant versatility in selecting the entry point for the biopsies because of the completeness of the CT image. A full 360 degree view of the patient is provided. All organs, including the bowel, are visualized, so that a variety of needle pathways can be chosen. It is possible to choose appropriate pathways to avoid specific organs or the bowel, if clinically indicated. Changing the body position of the patient may be advantageous for opening "windows" for instruments because of organ shifting or patient comfort. Finally, a wide variety of instruments can be used, ranging in size from a 22 gauge Chiba needle to a 14-guage Tru-cut needle. The ability to image high-density material accurately offers wide versatility, so that any type of instrument may be used in a procedure.

III. DISADVANTAGES OF CT-GUIDED PROCEDURES

- Cost
- Radiation
- Availability

CT guidance has a number of apparent disadvantages that are however, quite minimal in comparison to its advantages. Those to be considered include cost, radiation, and availability of equipment. Although, it is true that the cost is greater for CT than it is for other examinations, the cost savings of a CT biopsy, compared with alternative costs of surgery and/or hospitalization are remarkable.

IV. INDICATIONS FOR CT-GUIDED PROCEDURES

The indications for CT-guided procedures vary from institution to institution, depending on the expertise of the radiologists and the available imaging modalities.

Smaller lesions :

- Lesions in critical areas (hilum)
- Retroperitoneal and pelvic lesions
- For any lesion, the biopsy route of which needs avoidance of bowel loop and vasculature
- Immunocompromised patients
- Deep-seated lesions

Generally the important factors to consider are the visibility of the lesion on CT as compared with other modalities, the type of pathologic sample required, and the location of the lesion. Considering that the prime function of the guidance modality is to direct the needle to the lesion, visibility of the lesion is the most obvious factor. If a lesion is seen only on CT or much better on CT, then CT is the modality of choice. When lesions are small (ranging from 3 to 5 cm) and are located in critical areas, CT is again the preferred modality. Critical areas best suited for CT punctures include abnormalities adjacent to major vessels, the hilum of the spleen, and the mediastinum. CT should be used when avoidance of intestinal loops or vascular structures is important. When a large cutting needle biopsy is clinically indicated, CT is usually the modality of choice. Even though fluoroscopy or ultrasound can be used safely in some cases, CT is the best guidance modality because it eliminates the two most likely errors: (1) inappropriate biopsy of uninvolved organs (e.g. gall bladder, vessels), and (2) inappropriate biopsy of abnormalities with increased vascularity.

V. SOME BASIC RULES OF CT GUIDED BIOPSY

- Explain the procedure at length to the patient and relatives
- Try to keep the patient in good humour and psychologically comfortable
- Good local anesthesia at puncture site
- Allow patient to breathe (controlled frequent) with needle in position.
- Perform biopsy in most comfortable position to the patient, if possible.
- Interventional radiologist must be familiar with management of any complications, e.g. pneumothorax—aspirate air under CT and insert an intercostal drainage etc.

VI. BASIC STEPS

CT-guided biopsy is not a complicated procedure. It can be broken down into several basic steps.

1. The procedure is explained to the patient and informed consent is obtained.
2. Appropriate laboratory values are obtained. Most laboratory evaluations include prothrombin time, partial thromboplastin time and platelet count.
3. The scan is plotted. This process includes careful review of the patient's previous CT study to determine the optimal patient position, whether oral or intravenous contrast medium is indicated, and the appropriate level for the biopsy.
4. Premedication is given prior to the procedure, according to the merit of the case.
5. The patient should be positioned AP, prone, oblique or lateral according to pathology concerned, by padding or cushioning the patient. The scanogram and appropriate cross-sectional images are obtained through the selected area. An important consideration in scanning for a biopsy procedure is patient breathing. Clear instructions are essential so that each breath is as similar as possible. The breathing command should be given for each slice. As the needle is placed, the patient is again asked to suspend breathing.
6. The best location for needle entry is selected, and a metallic marker is placed on the skin with the localizer light on the CT scanner.
7. The scan is repeated to confirm the suitability of the selected entry location.
8. With the distance measurement on the CT system, the distance from the marker on the patient's skin to the lesion is measured. This measure determines the optimal depth and angle for needle placement.
9. The patient's skin is prepared according to aseptic procedure guidelines. A sterile drape is applied, a local anesthetic (lidocaine 1%) is administered and the biopsy needle is placed superficially.
10. The scan is repeated at the needle location as well as one slice above and one slice below the expected needle location until the tip of the needle is visualized. The needle tip is advanced or manipulated until the correct position is obtained.
11. If the CT images confirm the correct location of the needle, a tissue sample is taken and prepared according to laboratory protocols.
12. Post-procedure scans are taken at 10 mm slice thickness to identify complication such as pneumothorax or hematoma.

The features that make CT an excellent choice for guiding a needle biopsy are also beneficial in performing percutaneous abscess drainage. Fluid collections that respond most favourably to percutaneous abscess drainage are well defined, unilocular, free-flowing and accessible. Often abscess drainage is performed under less favourable conditions (e.g., fluid collection is multiloculated, composed of necrotic tissue, or poorly defined) if the patient is a poor surgical candidate. In general, the shortest, straightest access route to the collection is favoured. However, care should be taken to avoid major vessels, bowel loops, and the pleural space. After the needle is placed, a drainage catheter is kept in place; the collection is aspirated as completely as possible. Catheters are usually left to gravity drainage. When drainage is complete, the catheter is withdrawn gradually.

VII. PREPROCEDURAL STEPS

Patient consent and history

Before the procedure and the administration of any tranquilizer medication, it is important to discuss the procedure in depth with the patient. All details, including the rationale, medical alternatives, method of the procedure, sensations to be felt by the patient, and the post-procedural routine, should be mentioned. After this discussion the patient may sign the informed consent form and help confer about the need for any sedation. During this time, one should also inquire about any medication that may alter coagulation or platelet function.

Laboratory studies

For routine aspiration procedures on a patient with no history of coagulopathy or medication, partial thromboplastin time, prothrombin time, and platelet count studies should be adequate.

Site and trajectory selection

Several general comments about site selection and pathway are appropriate. It is important to decide on a pathway that traverses the least amount of uninvolved tissue and that is also the least precarious in terms of possible complications. The concept of using a shortest line to the trajectory is valid; the less liver, lung or other non-involved organ crossed the less the possibility for a problem. It is wise to avoid pathways that include major nerves or muscles. If a powerful muscle group contracts, a needle can be bent.

Skin preparation

Once the entrance site has been chosen, the skin is prepared with betadine and a local anesthetic agent such as xylocaine is administered. When infiltrating local anesthetic, completely infiltrate the pathway in two steps. In the first step, infiltrate the skin, subcutaneous tissue and the superficial muscles. After that level is reached, have the patient in suspended respiration and then infiltrate the local anesthetic down to and including the pleura, peritoneum, or the capsule of the liver.

VIII. SEDATION IN CT-GUIDED INTERVENTIONS

Conscious sedation is defined as a state of cortical depression in which the patient is tranquil and drowsy and may even close his or her eyes but may be able to respond to verbal commands. The protective reflex should be intact. Greater levels of anesthesia are used in vascular interventional procedures and with uncooperative patients, children and aged individuals.

IX. NEEDLE SELECTION

- Skinny needle (18-22)
- Cutting needle (14-20 G).
- Automated core biopsy system (biopsy gun).

A clinical decision about the biopsy must first be made according to the type of information sought by the attending physician from the pathologic sample. Generally, if a patient has a known malignancy and only a confirmation of metastases or recurrence is desired, an aspiration biopsy with a skinny needle is all that is required. If a patient has an unknown problem or if a question of a second malignancy exists, a large-cutting-needle biopsy is indicated. Only a sample with such a needle can accurately make the diagnosis of a lymphoma, benign tumor, or an unusual tumor. If a clinical decision is made to use a large needle, consideration of clinical, laboratory, anatomic and dynamic scan information should be made. Clinically, there must be no history of a coagulopathy, and the patient must not be on any type of medication that would impair coagulation or platelet function. Careful consideration of the anatomy, from a recent or current baseline CT obtained during the planning of the procedure, is appropriate. A large needle can be used if clear access is available to the organ of the abnormality. When tumors are seen as very vascular on CT, one should certainly avoid biopsy with cutting needles and should even use a gentle technique with aspiration needles. Any tumors or abnormality that shows considerable vascularity should only be biopsied carefully by an aspiration needle and not by a cutting needle.

Aspirating needles versus cutting needles

There has been some controversy about the diagnostic yields and the complication rates of aspiration needles and cutting needles. It is my opinion that both types of instruments can be used safely and effectively if appropriate techniques are used. As for the assertion that cytological results yield accurate results with all abnormalities, it is clearly not correct. While abundant evidence exists supporting the usefulness of the skinny needle for epithelial tumors, careful review of the literature results in an awareness that most authors recognize the problem of providing a definitive diagnosis for lymphomas, unusual tumors, or benign abnormalities.

Selection of aspiration needle

The larger the caliber of the aspiration needles the better the results. Also if the angle of the bevel is varied, the small angle provides the most diagnostic tissue. The bevel of the Chiba needle (25 degrees) actually provides the best sample.

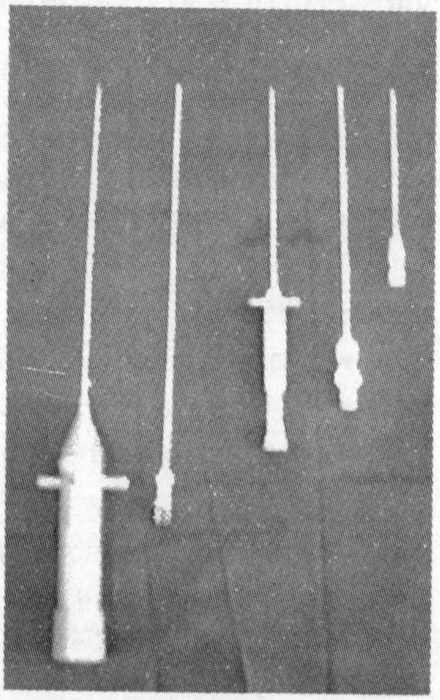

Fig. 25.1. Different types of needles : 1. Biopsy gun, 2. Chiba needle, 3. Tru-cut biopsy needle, 4. Bone biopsy needle (Osteocut), 5. Aspiration needle.

Choice of cutting needles

There are two basic types of cutting needles that can be used to obtain samples. They are available in a variety of sizes. The end-cutting Menghini needle and the side cutting Tru-cut needles are the prototypes of these devices. The Tru-cut needle may be preferred for almost all cutting biopsy procedure. Menghini may be preferred for tumors that are very hard, especially those within bone. The second circumstance is where the Menghini needle used is in deep-seated mass.

X. CLINICAL NEEDLE TECHNIQUES

There are basically four different placement techniques that can be used for needle aspiration :

- Single needle method – commonest
- Short cannula coaxial–lung biopsy, deep-seated abdominal masses.
- Long cannula coaxial method – uncommon
- Tandem needle method - rare pancreatic malignancies

Single needle method

With this method, the needle is placed in the skin and subcutaneous tissue and incremental adjustments are made. Adjustments are made with changes in the angulation and sequential scan. Once the correct angulation is achieved, the needle is inserted to the appropriate depth until the needle tip is at the proper location. This method is somewhat more difficult than the short cannula method because if the needle being used is long, the weight and length of the needle make it "hang". In such cases, the short length in the tissues will not support the weight of the needle, making determination of the angle before insertion into the tissues as difficult.

Short cannula coaxial method

This method is well suited for lung biopsies and small, deeply located masses in the abdomen. For this method, a 16-gauge 1½ inch hypodermic needle as the cannula and the 20 gauge Chiba needle for the aspiration needle may be recommended. For those who prefer a 22 gauage Chiba, an 18 gauge hypodermic can be used. The greatest advantage of this method is that the short guidance cannula predetermines the angle prior to the insertion of the aspiration needle. The angle of the guidance cannula, which is external to the body cavity, is adjusted until the trajectory is correct. Numerous adjustments in the angle can be made without injury to internal structures because the aspiration needle is not inserted until the correct angle is obtained. Once this is accomplished the aspiration needle is inserted and the only factor to contend with it is the distance to the lesion, which can be incrementally adjusted. The cannula can provide access for several repeat biopsies if desired. If one wishes to sample slightly different areas of a mass, the cannula can intentionally be deviated to guide the aspiration needle to different parts of the mass. The cannula (hypodermic needle) should only be inserted into the superficial structures without entering the body cavity. Too deep a placement could injure organs.

Long cannula coaxial method

This method uses a long guidance cannula, which is inserted to the depth of the lesion. The long cannula, which has a large diameter of 18 gauge or greater, is positioned with the single–needle method as noted above. The disadvantages are that a large needle is used to traverse the tissue, the single-needle method must be used, and the multiple aspirations are actually confined to a small area rather than being somewhat separate.

XI. ASPIRATION TECHNIQUE

After successful placement of the instrument within the lesion using any of the above methods, the following steps are taken. Ensure that the needle tip is definitely in the lesion and that circular and reciprocating motions are made during the application of suction. For best results, limit the reciprocating motion to about 1 to 2 cm distance. Try to keep at least 10 cc of suction applied during these motions. The most critical factor after removal of the sample is the pathologic fixation of the material obtained. After the sample has been removed it should be ejected onto a slide, and smear should be made with a second slide. Both slides should be quickly inserted into the appropriate fixative to prevent air drying.

Number of passes

It has been well documented that taking two passes for every procedure doubles the complication rate and only minimally increases the diagnostic yield.

Sample preparation

Perform the smear quickly in close proximity to the fixative to prevent drying, which can occur fast. Always flush the syringe and needle with fixative and send the fluid for tissue cell block.

XII. INSERTION OF CUTTING NEEDLE

The Menghini–type cutting needle

Advance the instrument against the lesion to be sampled and confirm the location next to the lesion. Then measure the depth of the desired sample and set any marker or mechanical stop appropriately. Apply suction and insert the needle to the desired depth.

Manual Tru–cut or side cutting needles

Insert the closed instrument to the edge of the lesion and confirm the position. Insert the inner stylet and reconfirm the position. To take the sample, hold the inner stylet stationary and advance the outer cannula over the stylet and remove the needle. Place the sample in the chosen tissue fixative and send it with appropriate information to the pathologist.

Automated side needle devices

Most of these are a permutation on the Tru-cut design but some are a refinement of a Menghini-type needle. There are three reasons to use such devices. First, as a routine these devices are easier to use and more consistently provide a high-quality sample. Second, in very obese patients, they clearly provide superior samples. It is very difficult to obtain a good sample using a manual device because of the friction or "drag" put on the cutting cannula when it is moved forward. Finally, when tumors are extremely hard, automated devices permit better recovery of samples because the firm tissue also produces a drag on the outer cannula. If the devices are too long or too heavy they do not adapt well to use with CT scanners. The best–suited devices have needles that are detachable from the gun. With these the needle is localized with the single–needle method and the mechanized portion is attached before taking the sample.

Angle or out-of–slice procedure

After one has mastered the straight or the in-slice method, one can learn to perform angled biopsies with the entrance site at one level and the target lesion at another level. This technique is most valuable for the sampling of lesions within the pelvis, below the iliac wing, and under the dome of the diaphragm, as well as in trying to avoid certain structures within the abdomen.

Localization of the needle tip

After insertion of the needle, one may occasionally have some difficulty in localizing the tip. There are several methods that can be used to solve this problem. The simplest method is to take a longitudinal scout and take an axial slice at the end. This is virtually foolproof and is the most expeditious. Another method, which can be used if the angle of the needle is slight, involves simply taking multiple scans in one direction until the end of the needle is reached. Many of the new scanners have a simple feature of a cluster scan consisting of three or more scans, which is well suited for this purpose. When the end of the needle is found, it will appear to have a square end and may have an artifact from the end. On occasion the end of the needle will not be "square" in appearance, but the end is easily appreciated by noting when the end is no longer seen on subsequent scans.

XIII. GENERAL COMPLICATIONS OF CT-GUIDED PROCEDURES

If proper CT techniques are used, the major causes of complications are limited to poor technique, lack of patient cooperation, undetected coagulopathy, or undiagnosed obstructive or diffuse interstitial processes in the lung.

- Usually cutting needle has comparatively higher complications rate than skinny needle.
- Organ insult with inflammation—pancreatitis, cholangitis
- Fistulae
- Needle tract seeding (?)
- Hemorrhage
- Pneumopthorax
- Vascular injury
- Infection
- Vasovagal reaction

Skinny–needle complications

The skinny needle is the safest instrument available but even this needle can produce complications in selected circumstances. Most complications have occurred when lesions have been very vascular or when numerous needle passes have been made.

Cutting–needle complications

With large needles one obviously has a greater probability of incurring many possible complications because a large "hole" is being produced. The new automated cutting devices are no safer than the standard Tru-cut needle.

Hemorrhage

The most likely potential risk during any biopsy procedure is the occurrence of bleeding. The vascularity of the pathologic lesion, as well as the anatomy, occurrence rate, and risk of bleeding are specific for each organ system. Obviously, to avoid complications one must ensure that a patient does not have any coagulopathy and that the laboratory values are within acceptable ranges.

Patient cooperation

The most critical factor in enhancing patient cooperation is adequate local anesthesia in the area of the biopsy. Local anesthesia should be administered down to the serosal surface of the organ (e.g. pleura, capsule). If this area is not anesthetized the patient may "jerk" at the time of insertion and produce a tear, bleed or pneumothorax. For those patients who are emotionally upset, administration of an appropriate hypnotic or sedative can be quite helpful.

Pyogenic contamination

Contamination of sterile areas is possible from either a cutaneous source or, if a loop of bowel is penetrated, an enteric source. If betadine is used for preparation of the skin, cutaneous contamination is improbable. Contamination from bowel can occur, depending on the immune status of the patient, the nature of the abnormality, the size of the pyogenic inoculum, and the virulence of the pathogens. It is true that an immunocompetent patient can tolerate spillage of a small amount of bacteria within the peritoneum, but the clearance of bacteria is impaired in certain circumstances. If bacteria are introduced into a fluid space, experimental data show that the effectiveness of bacteria "killing" is impaired because (1) "opsonization" of pyogens by antibodies and complement is less efficient in a fluid space, and (2) phagocyte-clearing activity is impaired in a fluid space. Moreover, an immunocompromised patient is obviously at a greater risk from pyogenic organisms. If the patient is known to be immunocompromised, avoid traversing colon or small bowel in all cases. Avoidance of bowel in any of the cases noted above can usually be achieved by changing the position of the patient; this may result in a "shifting" of the bowel that may open clear pathways for needle insertion.

Vasovagal and hysterical reactions

The vasovagal reaction is a sudden discharge of the parasympathetic vagal nerve, resulting in bradycardia, vasodilatation and hypotension. The patient should first be put in a Trendelenberg position to enhance venous return to the heart and cerebral blood flow. If the patient improves within 1 to 2 minutes, no other action need be taken. However, if the patient does not improve quickly, oxygen should be administered by nasal cannula and an appropriate dose of atropine, either intramuscularly or intravenously, should be administered. Urgent consultation with a resuscitation team is appropriate.

Tumour recurrence in needle pathway

Growth of residual tumor cells traced through needle pathways is a potential but fortunately rare problem. In reality, most tumors are inoperative when they are biopsied, but if there is a possibility of curative resection, a trajectory should be chosen that would permit resection of the needle track by the surgeon.

XIV. COMMON CT-GUIDED PROCEDURES

Diagnostic

- Fine needle aspiration cytology/culture sensitivity
- True cut biopsy

Therapeutic

- Tumour ablation—usually for hepatoma
- Lymphocoele
- Renal and liver cyst
- Pancreatic pseudocyst
- Abscess
- Percutaneous nephrostomy
- CT-guided nerve blocks
  (a) Celiac nerve block
  (b) Lumbar sympathectomy

Adjuncts to abscess drainage

1. Antibiotics—systemic antibiotics before and during drainage
2. Mucolytic agents to decrease viscosity, purulent material controversial
3. Fibrinolytic agent—urokinase to facilitate drainage of purulent material

XV. SUPPLIES FOR BIOPSY AND DRAINAGE PROCEDURES

Personnel protective equipment

- Face shields
- Sterile gowns
- Sterile gloves

Needles

- Spinal needles (18, 20, 22 gauge)
- Chiba (20, 22 gauge; 15, 20 cm)
- Trucut (14, 16, 18 guage)
- Automatic core biopsy system (biopsy gun) (22 guage, 20 gauge, 18 guage)

Surgical items

- Sterile 4 × 4 gauze sponges, sterile drape
- Sterile needles, sterile syringes, scalpel
- Betadine, 1% lidocaine
- Pigtail catheter (8, 10 French)
- Fascial dilators (6, 8, 10 French)
- Guide wires (0.025 m, 0. 038 J-tipped)
- Tubes/bottles for laboratory studies
- Formalin or nonbacteriostatic saline
- Albuminised glass slides
- Sutures (nylon or prolene)
- Drainage bag and connecting tubing

Others

- Metallic skin markers
- Skin marking pen

CHAPTER 27

An Overview of the Relevance and Future of CT

Computed tomography by the advent of spiral and multislice technology has dramaticaly improved in terms of image quality and speed. But in the coming years, the uses of CT will become more and more closely scrutinized as MRI becomes better, faster and cheaper. The radiation aspects of CT will also become more controversial. As of now it could be argued that all cranial cross-sectional studies, except those for acute trauma, acute subarachnoid hemorrhage or where there are known MRI contra-indications may be performed by MRI. CT is very usefull in detecting subtle calcifications. 3D CT is very usefull in craniostenosis and craniofacial trauma. Skull base and foraminal evaluation require CT. HRCT of temporal bones and floor of anterior cranial fossa are particularly usefull.

Similarly, for the spine, there are very few anatomical structures or lesions which are shown better by CT. Cervical disc herniations provide on exception; these lesions are still considered by most workers to be better depicted by CT myelography than MRI. The actual bony detail of the vertebrae and spinal canal is better shown by CT and thus CT may be preferred to show the exact extent of osseous degenerative conditions and lesions such as osteoid osteoma. However, these constitute a small percentage of referrals and MRI is generally the preferred option. Furthermore, the extended coverage with modern phased array coils provide MRI with yet further advantages.

A similar picture is emerging for musculoskeletal problems, for which MRI is nearly always the technique of choice. Those referrals where exact display of bone details is required are again exceptions. For example, depiction of a complex tibial plateau fracture is better performed by CT. Some workers argue that CT arthrography is better than plain MRI for certain problems in the shoulder joint . But generally the multiplanar capabilities and the better delineation of the soft tissues give MRI substantial advantages.

Within the chest, CT is still generally preferred. Although mediastinal lesions can now be well demonstrated by MRI, CT is usually quicker and simpler. Certainly for abnormalities within the lung parenchyma, high-resolution CT techniques provide unassailable detail. Although MRI can detect small pulmonary nodules, CT remains the preferred option in the detection of possible metastases and the characterization of other nodular lesions. MRI will eventually take over most cardiac imaging problems which cannot be solved by ultrasound.

For abdominal and pelvic lesions, the choice between CT and MRI is not clear-cut. Where the clinical questions concern just one anatomical region a strong case for MRI can be made. However, where a general survey of the whole abdomen is needed CT is still much to be preferred. In practice few MRI centres have much experience in thoracic and abdominal work; neurological and orthopaedic work tend to fill the available capacity.

Despite the exciting advances in MRI and despite of the radiation worries about CT, there will still be a large stage for CT over the next decade. Indeed it could be argued that MRI has provided the stimulus for the further advances in CT. Spiral CT will become the norm, resulting in a large increase in patient throughput. Costs might come down drastically. Image manipulation will become easier, thus 3D CT for aneurysms, fractures and other bony structures wiil become a routine. Whatever the future of CT brings in terms of instant 3D and interactive displays, automatic colour highlighting of tumours, etc, there will still be a need for an understanding of the principles of CT and the various methods of data acquisition. There will also continue to be a need for a close understanding of cross-sectional anatomy.

It is unlikely that there will be much further improvement in image quality of the standard axial images. Even though this might be technically possible, it is likely that a considerably larger radiation dose would be needed. Furthermore, any increase in the number of pixels per image (1024 × 1024 on many existing systems) would make data handling even more difficult. Multislice CT can be seen as a continuation of the exciting innovation introduced by spiral CT. Newer multislice CT will make imaging ultrafast and large volume coverage possible and it will have a major role in cardiac imaging. It may be possible to develop a cone beam area detector CT in the place of current multifan beam multi slice detector CT. Fusion of images generated from different imaging modalities such as MR, CT and PET showing advantages of both techniques may become very popular.